Ordering Information

The paperback sourcebooks listed below are published quarterly and can be ordered either by subscription or single copy.

Subscriptions cost $52.00 per year for institutions, agencies, and libraries. Individuals can subscribe at the special rate of $39.00 per year *if payment is by personal check.* (Note that the full rate of $52.00 applies if payment is by institutional check, even if the subscription is designated for an individual.) Standing orders are accepted.

Single copies are available at $12.95 when payment accompanies order. (California, New Jersey, New York, and Washington, D.C., residents please include appropriate sales tax.) For billed orders, cost per copy is $12.95 plus postage and handling.

Substantial discounts are offered to organizations and individuals wishing to purchase bulk quantities of Jossey-Bass sourcebooks. Please inquire.

Please note that these prices are for the academic year 1987–88 and are subject to change without notice. Also, some titles may be out of print and therefore not available for sale.

To ensure correct and prompt delivery, all orders must give either the *name of an individual* or an *official purchase order number.* Please submit your order as follows:

Subscriptions: specify series and year subscription is to begin.
Single Copies: specify sourcebook code (such as, MHS1) and first two words of title.

Mail orders for United States and Possessions, Latin America, Canada, Japan, Australia, and New Zealand to:
    Jossey-Bass Inc., Publishers
    433 California Street
    San Francisco, California 94104

Mail orders for all other parts of the world to:
    Jossey-Bass Limited
    28 Banner Street
    London EC1Y 8QE

New Directions for Mental Health Services Series
H. Richard Lamb, *Editor-in-Chief*

MHS1   *Alternatives to Acute Hospitalization,* H. Richard Lamb
MHS2   *Community Support Systems for the Long-Term Patient,* Leonard I. Stein
MHS3   *Mental Health Consultations in Community Settings,*
        Alexander S. Rogawski

Contents

Editor's Notes

The most seriously mentally ill are a neglected population. While they typically have profound needs, the services they require are provided by a confusing array of programs and agencies that are poorly coordinated and often competing. The bewildering distribution of responsibility among different levels of government and such varying providers as those of medical care, housing, and disability assistance almost guarantees significant gaps in service and a lack of accountability. The severely disabled inevitably depend on public services, but the public sector is too disorganized and demoralized to respond appropriately to the challenge. To solve the problem of providing adequate care for the chronically mentally ill, we need no less than a revitalization of public mental health services.

The first step in the revitalization of public mental health services is to understand the social and institutional processes of mental health care and how they have been shaped by historical factors and by our systems of government, law, and health and welfare entitlements. Mental health care is as much influenced by general social policy and culture as it is by policy decisions within the mental health specialty sector. All of the contributors to this volume are social scientists associated with the Institute for Health, Health Care Policy, and Aging Research at Rutgers University. The institute is committed to the study of severe mental illness and the broad social context of mental health care. Much of mental health research focuses on categorical issues viewed from the perspective of a single discipline. In contrast, the institute is dedicated to the interdisciplinary study of important health issues and seeks to understand the wide range of considerations essential to improving mental health services.

In the first chapter, I examine briefly how our current pattern of care has evolved and areas that offer promising opportunities for change. Gerald Grob, a historian at the institute, then reviews how mental health policy developed in the post–World War II period and describes the philosophical and political dialogue that contributed to these developments.

In Chapter Three, Allan Horwitz examines the help-seeking networks that bring patients into care or that pose obstacles. Sarah Rosenfield, in Chapter Four, explores how various components of community mental health programs can contribute to the quality of life of the severely mentally ill. Then, anthropologist Ann Dill examines the ways in which bureaucracy and the need for personal intimacy in client relationships affect the work of the case manager.

1

Perhaps the single largest obstacle to community care for the severely disabled is the lack of suitable housing. Carol Boyer, in Chapter Six, depicts the obstacles to solving this crucial problem. In the following chapter, Steven Crystal, a sociologist and former administrator of human services in New York City, and Edmund Dejowski, a clinical psychologist and lawyer, describe a range of protective services for patients who are unable to take responsibility for themselves.

The final three chapters deal with the broader political, economic, and legal contexts. Political scientist David Rochefort reviews the complex environment of policy formulation and implementation, while economist Jeffrey Rubin examines various approaches to the financing of mental health care, particularly in the public sector. In the last chapter, Alexander Brooks, a mental health legal scholar, explores the growing interest in and implications of outpatient commitment.

This sourcebook conveys the complexity of mental health services delivery and policy formulation. We hope it also introduces promising initiatives and suggests opportunities for improved care.

David Mechanic
Editor

David Mechanic is director of the Institute for Health, Health Care Policy, and Aging Research, university professor, and René Dubos Professor of behavioral sciences, Rutgers University.

Appropriate care for the most seriously mentally disabled will require an improved framework for public-sector services, Medicaid reforms, systems of managed care, and effective advocacy.

Evolution of Mental Health Services and Areas for Change

David Mechanic

Ideology and rhetoric played a major role in mental health policy and the evolution of the services systems in the post–World War II years (as Gerald Grob describes in Chapter Two). They helped shape perceptions of mental patients, views of how services should be organized and delivered, and the agenda for public policy. It was commonly assumed that mental illness was a relatively simple continuum from mild to severe and predominantly a product of socioenvironmental forces (Mechanic, 1980). From this assumption followed the optimistic view that early and appropriate intervention could prevent serious mental illness and even cure schizophrenia and other psychoses. These simplistic and untested assumptions (and many others concerning labeling processes, community integration of deinstitutionalized patients, and the potential of psychodynamic interventions) contributed to the confusion and neglect that continues to affect the care of the most seriously disabled long-term patients.

The mental health sector has a long history of cycles of optimism and despair (Grob, 1983). The pessimism of the 1980s is in part a reaction to the inflated promises of the 1960s. A number of influences have contributed to this pessimism: changes in the general public perception of the prospects for reform; economic problems and the growth of government deficits; the changing dynamics of health care organization and

D. Mechanic (ed.). *Improving Mental Health Services: What the Social Sciences Can Tell Us.*
New Directions for Mental Health Services, no. 36. San Francisco: Jossey-Bass, 1987.

pressures to contain costs; the medicalization of psychiatry, its focus on biological models, and diminished interest in social psychiatry; and the seemingly massive population of poorly served chronically mentally ill in communities.

This pessimism in turn creates exaggerated and nonconstructive public perceptions. For example, the mental health sector is increasingly held accountable for conditions outside its control (Mechanic, 1987). Along with policies of deinstitutionalization, this sector is increasingly blamed for the large number of patients without proper care, for the disturbing growth of homelessness, and for a mental health system in shambles. Serious reform depends on a clear separation of real problems from rhetoric and on a well-formulated strategy of response.

Deinstitutionalization and the Mentally Ill in the Community

Although there has been a large reduction in public mental health hospital beds as well as total inpatient days from all sources of inpatient psychiatric care (Kiesler and Sibulkin, 1983), deinstitutionalization alone cannot explain the massive numbers of seriously ill mental patients in communities. More important is the current population age structure and the numbers of persons in varying age groups who risk experiencing mental illness. The baby boom cohorts have now reached ages of high incidence of mental disorder, resulting in large aggregate numbers of seriously mentally ill youth. Moreover, disorders such as schizophrenia are often most troublesome and disruptive in early stages of the illness career, when other developmental problems are common (Harding and others, 1986; Clausen, Pfeffer, and Huffine, 1982; Bleuler, 1978; Ciompi, 1980), and this pattern increases the impact of mentally ill youth on the community. Finally, we are now dealing with cohorts of youth who are more likely than earlier cohorts to have assimilated antipsychiatric and libertarian ideologies, making them more difficult to treat and manage by conventional approaches (Schwartz and Goldfinger, 1981; Sheets, Prevost, and Reihman, 1982).

Thus, the problems of community care for young schizophrenics would be with us, although to a somewhat lesser degree, even if we had not eliminated a single hospital bed. Moreover, overwhelming evidence suggests that, for most of the severely mentally ill, long-term institutional care is neither beneficial nor cost effective (Stein and Test, 1980; Weisbrod, Test, and Stein, 1980; New South Wales Department of Health, 1983; Kiesler and Sibulkin, 1987).

Homelessness and Mental Illness

A related misconception is that prevalent homelessness is in large part caused by deinstitutionalization and that the problems of the homeless mentally ill are fundamentally different from those who have suitable shelter. The determinants of homelessness are not fully understood nor is its permanence clear. Many factors contribute, including a diminishing supply of low-cost housing in many cities as well as rising housing costs in relation to reduced general assistance and welfare payments. All homeless people face a complex and interrelated array of problems and needs that are economic, social, and medical (Rossi, Wright, Fisher, and Willis, 1987; Bassuk, 1984; U.S. General Accounting Office, 1985). Physical and psychiatric disability exacerbate the problems, but these disabilities are probably not fundamental causes of homelessness.

To observe that many of the homeless have serious psychiatric disabilities is quite different from suggesting that homelessness is a product of deinstitutionalization. Estimates of mental illness among the homeless vary widely from one study to another, but a fair guess is that one-fifth to one-third may have significant psychiatric disability beyond the distress, anxiety, and depression reasonably resulting from being indigent and without shelter. The most careful study of homelessness (in Chicago) found that 25 percent of the homeless located in a thorough survey of streets and shelters reported having at some time been in a psychiatric unit for a stay of more than forty-eight hours, and half of the homeless reported significant depressive symptoms (Rossi, Wright, Fisher, and Willis, 1987). Many had been jailed or had spent time in a detoxification unit. In short, this is a population of great need, but it is essential not to confuse causes or the significant policy issues. Nor is there reason to assume that most of the homeless who are mentally ill are less treatable than others once adequate shelter and supervision have been provided.

The Importance of Rehabilitation

The large numbers of schizophrenics, drug-abusing youth, and others with chronic debilitating disorders, so evident in large cities, require approaches very different from those prevalent in earlier decades. The appropriate model is rehabilitation, and its goals must be maintenance of function and quality of life (Shepherd, 1984; Watts and Bennett, 1983). Moreover, services must be oriented to longitudinal and not episodic care, and the overall approach must be sensitive but aggressive and not dependent on compliant client help seeking.

Rehabilitation is based on the assumption of an irreversible limitation, whether defined by a disease process or a handicap, and seeks to maximize function by preventing secondary disabilities and assisting patients to cope constructively with their limitations. The emphasis is on ensuring that basic needs, such as shelter, psychiatric and medical care, and subsistence, are satisfied and that social adjustment is facilitated by providing a reasonable level of activity, enhanced coping skills, and strengthened social supports (Wing, 1978). Psychiatric care is directed at minimizing psychotic symptoms, while other services are directed at bolstering living skills, self-esteem, and satisfaction. This is not to suggest that rehabilitation is easy; the difficult course of serious mental illness taxes morale and patience. The challenge is to build a mental health services system that ensures that these needs are addressed with defined populations of patients on a long-term basis and that mental health professionals themselves have the tools and supportive structures necessary for undertaking the required tasks (Mechanic, 1986a, 1987).

The Evolution of the Mental Health Services System

Mental health services now involve a complex mix among federal, state, and private resources, general and psychiatric hospitals, public and private institutions and programs, varying mental health providers, and hundreds of therapeutic interventions. The field is strongly influenced by financing streams, reimbursement rules, and organizational alignments. The problems treated range from desire for self-actualization and difficulties in everyday living to profound and persistent illnesses and disabilities. But shaping a system that makes sense for the most seriously mentally ill and that is responsive to those with lesser difficulties as well requires clear identification of the forces at work. These are only briefly noted here, but the discussion serves as a necessary basis for identifying important areas for change.

Changes in Insurance Coverage. In recent decades there has been an impressive growth of insurance for inpatient psychiatric care (Brady, Sharfstein, and Muszynski, 1986). By 1984 almost all firms above a minimum size provided employee inpatient coverage, and in about half the cases it was offered on the same basis as any other illness. Almost all firms also provided psychiatric outpatient coverage, but less than onetenth provided it on a basis comparable to other illnesses. Common restrictions are high coinsurance (typically 50 percent) and low dollar limits. Outpatient benefits are even more restricted in Medicare and other public programs. Existing patterns of insurance clearly provide incentives to inpatient care, and little opportunity to trade off such expenditures against outpatient treatment. The importance of insurance coverage is reflected in the fact that in 1984 there were almost 1.7 million discharges from short-stay hospitals with a primary mental illness diagnosis and an average length of stay of approximately twelve days (Dennison, 1985).

Patients with broad insurance coverage typically are treated in the private and voluntary acute care hospital sector, and those who exhaust their coverage or who are uninsured typically receive their care from public hospitals. Even those with Medicaid coverage are most commonly served by nonprofit institutions, but the filtering process brings the most chronic and intractable cases to the public sector. Inevitably the long-term chronically ill depend on the integrity of public mental health services, and the financing and organization of the public sector is crucial to a viable system of care. Understanding the current state of the public system requires some appreciation of its evolution in the past thirty years.

The Move Toward Deinstitutionalization. In 1955, when the number of mental patients in public institutions peaked at 560,000, the hospital played a dual role. With its relatively meager resources, it gave whatever acute care it could to new arrivals and also provided custodial care to a large residual population of long-term patients. Resources were directed to acute patients, and most returned to the community after a few months. The longer the patient remained, the greater the probability of neglect, and there was a deep sense of hopelessness about these patients (Mechanic, 1978b). The introduction of neuroleptics in the mid 1950s alleviated the most bizarre manifestations of psychosis and influenced the hope and confidence of administrators, caretakers, and families about community residence. This hope, allied with the emerging ideology of community care, a strong critique of the mental hospital, and a vigorous civil liberties movement on behalf of patients' rights, led to a desire for large-scale deinstitutionalization, but, in fact, the reduction of mental hospital populations proceeded at a modest average rate of 1.5 percent per year between 1955 and 1965 (Gronfein, 1985).

A major barrier during those years was the difficulty of relocating patients, and it was only with the welfare reforms of the 1960s and the expansion of medical and disability programs that a substantial reduction of hospital beds became possible. Medicaid stimulated the growth of the nursing home sector, provided an alternative placement for the demented patient as well as others, and gave states an opportunity to shift costs to the federal government. Social Security Disability Insurance (SSDI) and Supplemental Security Insurance (SSI) provided income that supported residence in board-and-care facilities and made it easier for families to cope with the economic burdens of having mentally ill members in the community. Between 1966 and 1980, inpatients in public mental hospitals fell by an average of 6 percent a year (Gronfein, 1985).

Change and State Mental Health Systems

The reduction of inpatient beds allowed many states to transform their mental hospitals into acute care institutions, and, by 1982, the average state hospital had 529 inpatients, 807 employees, and average expenses per patient of $31,000 (Dolan, 1986). Most states continue to focus their mental health funds on institutions because of their commitments to

8

maintain hospital improvements relevant to increased scrutiny by the public and the courts, because of the political pressures of hospital employees and communities that depend on the financing of hospitals, and because states are reluctant to take on new community commitments during a time of fiscal restraint. Approximately two-thirds of state expenditures continue to support state hospitals, although there is considerable state variation (National Institute of Mental Health, 1985). A major challenge is to fit the state hospitals and psychiatric inpatient units into a system of care that balances and integrates both inpatient and outpatient services.

The level of available resources is important, but the quality of state mental health systems depends even more on the structure of financing and organization. There is extraordinary variation among states in the extent to which their systems of care are institutionally based. In Wisconsin, for example, which historically had a unique system of county mental hospitals, state financing schemes now give local government powerful incentives to assess trade-offs between community and inpatient care and to seek alternatives to hospitalization (Stein and Ganser, 1983). This has facilitated the innovative Program of Assertive Community Treatment (PACT) model in Dane County and its dissemination (Stein and Test, 1985), but, even with a favorable financial structure, the results throughout the state have been uneven. Many factors continue to play a role: leadership; community attitudes; entrenched interest groups; competing agencies and professionals; and a conservative stance toward change (Mechanic, 1978a).

The problems of change are more difficult in states with large well-established hospital systems, communities dependent on hospitals, and well-organized and unionized employees. Such systems require transition strategies that increase the funds following the patient on a graduated basis, that guarantee the stability and integrity of care in public hospitals over some reasonable period of time so intelligent planning can accompany the staging of change, and that facilitate working closely with unions and employees in programs of scheduled attrition and retraining. Outside stimuli such as litigation and court scrutiny, if applied intelligently, can help move the process forward, and strong leadership is essential for the delicate negotiations that are required with threatened segments of the community. Active involvement of groups representing the National Alliance for the Mentally Ill (NAMI) and other community advocates can help if they work cooperatively. The goal is to avoid polarization and to develop procedures that divert inappropriate admissions to community care but that initiate intensive discharge planning soon after the patient enters the hospital.

The debate over hospital versus community care is strongly ideological, often acrimonious, and rarely constructive. Hospital care will continue to play an important part in the care of serious mental illness, and some segment of patients will require long-term refuge either for their own benefit or for the protection of others (Gudeman and Shore, 1984). The focus of change in state mental health systems should be on the role of the hospital in a balanced system of care and on ways of ensuring high-quality care.

In many states, hospitals have valuable resources in the form of land and unused buildings. Some hospital systems have been innovative in using these resources to integrate the hospital into a broader environment (Dolan, 1986). These assets could also be used to diversify the environment on hospital grounds, to create new opportunities for patient habituation and vocational rehabilitation, and to generate new income for mental health services.

The Problem of the Uninsured and Medicaid Reform

The mental health services system has largely been shaped by such outside forces as insurance entitlements and welfare policies. For example, the future of care for the severely mentally ill will depend more on how the nation attacks the massive problem of the 37 million uninsured (Mechanic, 1986b; Bazzoli, 1986), how it modifies Medicaid, and how it handles SSDI, SSI, and housing issues than on areas more specifically related to mental illness. I will describe here the insurance issues; the housing and disability issues are addressed elsewhere in this sourcebook.

The use of mental health services is highly related to insurance coverage. In the Rand Health Experiment (a $100 million controlled experiment in which patients were randomized into varying coinsurance schemes), there were fourfold variations among different coinsurance groups in the use of mental health services (Keeler and others, 1986). Those with 50 percent coinsurance and no limits on cost sharing spent only two-fifths as much as those with no coinsurance. This response is much greater than is typically the case in general medical services (Ellis and McGuire, 1986). Coinsurance for mental health care primarily affects the number of episodes of treatment and much less the duration and intensity of care once a person enters treatment.

Research on the insured only begins to suggest the magnitude of the problem for persons with no insurance or those covered by Medicaid with its limitations in benefits and low levels of reimbursement for providers. Moreover, the Medicaid program has not expanded in the 1980s in response to the increase in poverty; it covers less than half of those who meet federal poverty standards (Curtis, 1986). Mentally ill persons above the poverty standard who are not covered by group insurance may have difficulty in gaining access to individual insurance at an affordable rate. An important idea of health insurance was to pool risk across large populations, but, in the current context of cost consciousness, more health plans are adopting risk-rating approaches that increase premiums for persons with a history of mental health treatment or exclude them entirely.

In the long run, solving the problems of the uninsured must be part of a larger health insurance framework that rededicates our society to the principle that medical care should be available in relation to need and not be rationed by age, race, income, region, or condition. A more fair and adequate insurance structure would go a long way toward improving access to care and services for all of the mentally ill. Under the current system, however, the poor and the most severely disabled patients are the least likely to have this access. To improve their plight, we must address the issue of Medicaid reforms and systems of managed care appropriate to their special needs.

At the federal level, Medicaid is the largest and most important program affecting the severely mentally disabled. While not applicable to the care of persons aged twenty-one to sixty-four in public institutions, Medicaid nevertheless accounted for expenditures of $991 million in state and county mental hospitals in 1983 (Reddick, Witkin, Atay, and Manderscheid, 1986) and pays for much psychiatric inpatient care in nonfederal general hospitals and private hospitals (National Institute of Mental Health, 1985). In 1980, Medicaid was the expected principal source of payment for 1.9 million inpatient days in nonfederal general hospitals and private psychiatric hospitals (National Institute of Mental Health, 1985).

Because there is typically little capacity to track the mentally ill through the services system, patients having an exacerbation of symptoms come or are brought to emergency rooms where they are commonly seen by professionals who do not know them. There is a strong bias toward admission in such circumstances. In a well-managed system with appropriate patient tracking, many of these expensive admissions could be prevented.

At present, there are limited incentives to prevent hospitalization, and there may be pressures to fill vacant beds. Medicaid reforms that would reallocate hospital savings to community programs offering managed care would provide the types of incentives necessary (Aiken, Somers, and Shore, 1986). Another way to create a balanced system would be to pool the expected inpatient and outpatient Medicaid contributions under the control of a single accountable entity that has responsibility for a defined population of mentally ill persons. Capturing these funds would allow greater flexibility in care decisions as well as the resources necessary to develop service components and hire appropriate personnel. Various funding sources, including state allocations to local government, local resources, and Medicaid, could be managed in the same way to develop a full range of integrated services.

The Importance of Mental Health Advocacy

Even when the financial and organizational framework is well conceived, human services systems require high levels of discretion and are not easily managed (Mechanic, 1974, 1976). They are susceptible to the vagaries of local political climates, depend substantially on the leadership qualities and interpersonal skills of mental health administrators, and require complex intraorganizational alignments at varying levels of political jurisdiction and across sectors with different and sometimes conflicting cultures. It takes no anthropologist to comprehend the distance one travels in systems of assumptions as one moves across sectors involving community mental health centers, the police, housing authorities, and welfare administrators. Problems are compounded by the stigma associated with psychotic illness, substance abuse, and bizarre behavior in public settings and by the ways mass media conceptualize and communicate these problems to a concerned public.

Mental health has always had sporadic and relatively weak advocacy. The reasons need no recounting, but in recent years vigorous new advocacy groups have emerged, particularly NAMI. Competing groups seem more willing to form useful coalitions, and public leaders more openly acknowledge mental illness in their families. This advocacy is an important new national resource and, if directed wisely, can be a significant factor in future policy. In the final analysis, whatever the quality of our knowledge or technical studies, health policy making is a political process that depends on the sophistication, influence, and aggressiveness of interested groups. Mental health, like health in general, is big business, in which many groups have an important stake. Mental health advocacy, particularly for the most severely disabled, is still a fragile activity, but its entry on the scene offers new possibilities for revitalizing community systems of care.

References

Aiken, L. H., Somers, S. A., and Shore, M. F. "Private Foundations in Health Affairs: A Case Study of the Development of a National Initiative for the Chronically Mentally Ill." *American Psychologist,* 1986, *41,* 1290-1295.

Bassuk, E. "The Homeless Problem." *Scientific American,* 1984, *251,* 40-45.

Bazzoli, G. J. "Health Care for the Indigent: Overview of Critical Issues." *Health Services Research,* 1986, *21,* 353-393.

Bleuler, M. *The Schizophrenic Disorders: Long-Term Patient and Family Studies.* (S. M. Clemens, trans.) New Haven, Conn.: Yale University Press, 1978.

Brady, J., Sharfstein, S. S., and Muszynski, I. L., Jr. "Trends in Private Insurance Coverage for Mental Illness." *The American Journal of Psychiatry,* 1986, *143,* 1276-1279.

Ciompi, L. "Natural History of Schizophrenia in the Long Term." *British Journal of Psychiatry,* 1980, *136,* 413-420.

12

Clausen, J. A., Pfeffer, N. G., and Huffine, C. L. "Help Seeking in Severe Mental Illness." In D. Mechanic (ed.), *Symptoms, Illness Behavior, and Help Seeking.* New Brunswick, N.J.: Rutgers University Press, 1982.

Curtis, R. "The Role of State Governments in Assuring Access to Care." *Inquiry,* 1986, *23,* 277-285.

Dennison, C. F. "1984 Summary: National Discharge Survey." *Advanced Data from Vital and Health Statistics,* no. 112. Hyattsville, Md.: National Center for Health Statistics, 1985.

Dolan, L. W. *Recent Trends in the Evolution of State Psychiatric Hospital Systems.* New Brunswick, N.J.: Rutgers-Princeton Program in Mental Health Research, 1986.

Ellis, R. P., and McGuire, T. G. "Cost Sharing and Patterns of Mental Health Care Utilization." *The Journal of Human Resources,* 1986, *21,* 359-379.

Grob, G. N. *Mental Illness and American Society: 1875-1940.* Princeton, N.J.: Princeton University Press, 1983.

Gronfein, W. "Incentives and Intentions in Mental Health Policy: A Comparison of the Medicaid and Community Mental Health Programs." *Journal of Health and Social Behavior,* 1985, *26,* 192-206.

Gudeman, J. E., and Shore, M. F. "Beyond Deinstitutionalization: A New Class of Facilities for the Mentally Ill." *New England Journal of Medicine,* 1984, *311,* 832-836.

Harding, C. M., Brooks, G. W., Ashikaga, T., Strauss, J. S., and Breier, A. *The Vermont Longitudinal Study, II: Long-Term Outcome for DSM-III Schizophrenia.* New Haven, Conn.: Department of Psychiatry, Yale University School of Medicine, 1986.

Keeler, E. B., Wells, K. B., Manning, W. G., Rumpel, J. D., and Hanley, J. M. *The Demand for Episodes of Mental Health Services.* Santa Monica, Calif.: Rand Corporation, 1986.

Kiesler, C. A., and Sibulkin, A. E. "Proportion of Inpatient Days for Mental Disorders: 1969-1978." *Hospital and Community Psychiatry,* 1983, *34,* 606-611.

Kiesler, C. A., and Sibulkin, A. E. *Mental Hospitals: Myths and Facts About a National Crisis.* Newbury Park, Calif.: Sage, 1987.

Mechanic, D. *Politics, Medicine, and Social Science.* New York: Wiley-Interscience, 1974.

Mechanic, D. *The Growth of Bureaucratic Medicine.* New York: Wiley-Interscience, 1976.

Mechanic, D. "Alternatives to Mental Hospital Treatment: A Sociological Perspective." In L. I. Stein, and M. A. Test (eds.), *Alternatives to Mental Hospital Treatment.* New York: Plenum, 1978a.

Mechanic, D. *Medical Sociology.* (2nd ed.) New York: Free Press, 1978b.

Mechanic, D. *Mental Health and Social Policy.* (Rev. ed.) Englewood Cliffs, N.J.: Prentice-Hall, 1980.

Mechanic, D. "The Challenge of Chronic Mental Illness: A Retrospective and Prospective View." *Hospital and Community Psychiatry,* 1986a, *37* (9), 891-896.

Mechanic, D. "Health Care for the Poor: Some Policy Alternatives." *Journal of Family Practice,* 1986b, *22,* 283-289.

Mechanic, D. "Correcting Misconceptions in Mental Health Policy: Strategies for Improved Care of the Seriously Mentally Ill." *Milbank Memorial Fund Quarterly,* 1987, *65* (2), 203-230.

National Institute of Mental Health. *Mental Health, United States, 1985.* Washington, D.C.: U.S. Government Printing Office, 1985.

New South Wales Department of Health. *Psychiatric Hospital Versus Community*

Treatment: A Controlled Study. Sydney, Australia: New South Wales Department of Health, 1983.

Reddick, R. W., Witkin, M. J., Atay, J. E., and Manderscheid, R. W. *Specialty Mental Health Organizations, United States, 1983–84.* Rockville, Md.: National Institute of Mental Health, 1986.

Rossi, P. H., Wright, J. D., Fisher, G. A., and Willis, G. "The Urban Homeless: Estimating Composition and Size." *Science,* 1987, *235,* 1336–1341.

Schwartz, S., and Goldfinger, S. "The New Chronic Patient: Clinical Characteristics of an Emerging Subgroup." *Hospital and Community Psychiatry,* 1981, *32,* 470–474.

Sheets, J., Prevost, J., and Reihman, J. "Young Adult Chronic Patients: Three Hypothesized Subgroups." *Hospital and Community Psychiatry,* 1982, *33,* 197–202.

Shepherd, G. *Institutional Care and Rehabilitation.* New York: Longman, 1984.

Stein, L., and Ganser, L. J. *Wisconsin's System for Funding Mental Health Services.* In J. A. Talbott (ed.), *Unified Mental Health Systems: Utopia Unrealized.* New Directions for Mental Health Services, no. 18. San Francisco: Jossey-Bass, 1983.

Stein, L. I., and Test, M. A. "Alternatives to Mental Hospital Treatment II: Social Cost." *Archives of General Psychiatry,* 1980, *37,* 409–412.

Stein, L. I., and Test, M. A. (eds.). *The Training in Community Living Model: A Decade of Experience.* New Directions for Mental Health Services, no. 26. San Francisco: Jossey-Bass, 1985.

U.S. General Accounting Office. *Homelessness: A Complex Problem and the Federal Response.* Washington, D.C.: U.S. General Accounting Office, 1985.

Watts, F. N., and Bennett, D. H. (eds.). *Theory and Practice of Psychiatric Rehabilitation.* New York: Wiley, 1983.

Weisbrod, B. A., Test, M. A., and Stein, L. I. "Alternatives to Mental Hospital Treatment II: Economic Benefit-Cost Analysis." *Archives of General Psychiatry,* 1980, *37,* 400–402.

Wing, J. K. *Reasoning About Madness.* Oxford: Oxford University Press, 1978.

David Mechanic is director of the Institute for Health, Health Care Policy, and Aging Research, university professor, and René Dubos Professor of behavioral sciences, Rutgers University.

*Between 1940 and 1963 mental health policy in the United
States underwent a fundamental change as the legitimacy of
institutional care was undermined by individuals and groups
committed to an environmentalist psychodynamic psychiatry
and to community-oriented programs.*

Mental Health Policy in Post-World War II America

Gerald N. Grob

On the eve of World War II, the framework of mental health policy
appeared stable. At its center was a system of public mental hospitals,
which were responsible for providing both treatment and care for mentally ill persons, regardless of their ability to pay the high costs associated
with protracted hospitalization. In 1940 such hospitals had a resident
population of about 410,000; an additional 59,000 patients were in Veterans Administration, county, and city institutions. As a group, public
institutions cared for nearly 98 percent of all institutionalized patients. A
substantial percentage of each state budget was devoted to the institutional care and treatment of the mentally ill. Although disagreements
over details of policy and quality of facilities persisted, there was little
questioning of the idea that the mentally ill should receive care and
treatment in mental hospitals. Correspondingly, American psychiatry
was an institutional specialty; more than two-thirds of the members of
the American Psychiatric Association (APA) practiced in public institutions as late as 1940.

Within two short decades, however, the consensus on mental
health policy virtually vanished. By the 1960s the legitimacy of institutional care and treatment was under attack. Activists promoted a new
policy whose goal was to provide care and treatment in the community

D. Mechanic (ed.). *Improving Mental Health Services: What the Social Sciences Can Tell Us.*
New Directions for Mental Health Services, no. 36. San Francisco: Jossey-Bass, 1987.

rather than in the mental hospital. Indeed, contemporaries often referred to a third or fourth "psychiatric revolution" equal in significance to the first "revolution" when Philippe Pinel allegedly broke the chains of Parisian lunatics in 1793. The new policy, in short, assumed the virtual end of traditional mental hospitals and the creation in their place of community alternatives.

What elements shaped the transformation of public policy between the 1940s and 1960s? The answer to this question is neither simple nor straightforward. Many answers provided by contemporary participants reflect personal ideological commitments as well as a desire to legitimate new policy departures. The passage of time and the dimunition of passions, however, provide an opportunity to analyze some of these elements as well as some of the anticipated and unanticipated results.

Precursors of Change

The changes that occurred in mental health policies after 1945 were linked to earlier developments. Of major significance was the change in the composition of the patient population of mental hospitals after 1890. Throughout the nineteenth century, patient populations were made up largely of acute cases institutionalized for less than twelve months. Elderly individuals were rarely sent to mental institutions. Between 1890 and 1940, however, the proportion of long-term chronic patients increased dramatically, and acute admissions declined proportionately. By 1923 more than half of all patients had been institutionalized for five years or more. The bulk of chronic patients were elderly or suffered from psychiatric illnesses associated with a somatic etiology (such as paresis). Consequently, mental hospitals provided custodial long-term care for a variety of dependent persons who were unable to survive without assistance. This overwhelmingly chronic population, in turn, contributed to the creation of a depressing internal institutional environment that appeared to have few redeeming qualities.

As the patient population of mental hospitals changed, the hospitals' links with psychiatry weakened, since psychiatrists clearly preferred a therapeutic to a custodial role. Moreover, the rise of modern "scientific" medicine stimulated psychiatrists in the prewar decades to redefine concepts of mental disease and therapeutic interventions. In so doing, they implicitly posited a conflict between the mental hospital with its custodial role and the imperatives of modern psychiatry.

Generally speaking, the traditional psychiatric model of disease was based on the assumption that there was a sharp distinction between health and disease. The presence of mental disease was indicated by dramatic behavioral and somatic signs that deviated from the prior normal behavior of that individual in fundamental ways. By the turn of the century, however, such representative figures as Sigmund Freud in Europe and Adolf Meyer in the United States had begun to argue that behavior occurred along a continuum that commenced with the normal and concluded with the abnormal, thus blurring the demarcation between health and disease. Admittedly, the new psychodynamic psychiatry (as it was often called) rejected neither the conventional belief that mental disease was a somatic illness nor somatic therapies. Nevertheless, its implications were of major importance. If there was a continuum from the normal to the abnormal, then the possibility existed that, before the process had run its course, psychiatric interventions in a noninstitutional setting could alter the outcome. Hence, early treatment in community facilities might prevent the onset of the severe mental diseases that required institutionalization. By the 1920s and 1930s, signs of modest change were already evident: Some psychiatrists were affiliated with child guidance community clinics; some were involved with the mental hygiene movement; and some attempted to apply psychoanalytic principles to the practice of psychiatry. The majority, however, still clung to their traditional base in mental hospitals.

The Impact of the War

Before 1940 the new psychodynamic psychiatry grew at a slow pace. The specialty was as yet preoccupied with the severe mental illnesses. World War II, however, proved to be a crucial catalyst. Wartime experiences seemed to provide conclusive evidence that the principles of psychodynamic psychiatry, when linked with new policies and institutions, had the possibility of revolutionizing the ways in which society perceived of and dealt with the mentally ill.

The initial involvement of psychiatrists in the war was with the selective service. Their role was to help identify, in advance, individuals unqualified for military service because of neuropsychiatric problems. The assumption underlying screening, of course, was that knowledge of personality and background could be used to predict predisposition to mental disorders. Mass screening, however, proved far more effective in theory than in practice; evidence that available techniques possessed predictive reliability was lacking. Moreover, military authorities were concerned about maximizing manpower resources; the rejection of 1,750,000 men for neuropsychiatric reasons aroused considerable anger.

The difficulties of screening, however, were soon eclipsed by the problems arising out of breakdowns among military personnel. Some exhibited psychological symptoms after a brief encounter with the rigors of military life; some on experiencing the threat of danger when they arrived in a war zone; and some broke down after prolonged exposure to life-threatening combat situations. As early as 1942, evidence mounted that the prolonged stress associated with warfare led to mental break-downs even among those who had manifested no prior symptomatology. The results of the Guadalcanal and North Africa campaigns seemed to confirm the belief that environmental stress played the major role in the etiology of mental maladjustment and that greater attention had to be given to the neuroses (as compared with the traditional concern with the psychoses). Fascination with the neuroses, in turn, presaged a far greater interest in the role of social and environmental factors. Indeed, William C. Menninger (chief of the army's neuropsychiatric division) emphasized that the "history or the personality makeup or the internal psychodynamic stresses" were less important in the adjustment process than "the force of factors in the environment which supported or dis-rupted the individual" (Menninger, 1946).

If the rigors of military life and the stress of combat—not the structure of personality—contributed to mental breakdown, then it fol-lowed that careful and intelligent planning could reduce the numbers of psychological casualties. Hence, to minimize the dangers of "combat exhaustion," psychiatrists urged limitations on the time soldiers were kept in actual combat (in other words, fixed tours of duty); measures to promote group cohesion; and regular rest periods. They insisted that the neuroses of war were amenable to such treatments as brief psychotherapy and narcosynthesis. The success in returning servicemen who had experi-enced psychological problems to active duty reinforced a spirit of thera-peutic activism, which was subsequently carried back to civilian life.

The belief that environmental stress contributed to mental mal-adjustment enhanced the view that human interventions could alter psy-chological outcomes. That so many men had been rejected for military service because of neuropsychiatric disorders suggested that the mental illnesses were far more serious a public health problem than was gener-ally recognized. The lessons of the conflict thus seemed to confirm the earlier experiences of World War I and the principles of psychodynamic and psychoanalytic psychiatry. The claim that environmental factors played a major role in the etiology of mental disorders was to be reiter-ated over and over by a generation of psychiatrists who served in the military during World War II and assumed leadership roles in the post-war era. The concept that there was a smooth continuum from health to disease became an article of faith that justified psychiatric interventions well before the onset of the acute stage of any of the mental illnesses.

The psychiatric lessons gleaned from wartime experiences had significant policy implications. The greatest successes in treating soldiers with psychological symptoms occurred at the battalion aid-station level. Conversely, the therapeutic success rate declined in rear echelon units. A logical conclusion followed: Treatment in civilian life, as in the military, had to be provided in a family and community setting rather than in a remote or isolated institution. The implication for psychiatry was clear: community and private practice would replace institutional employment.

Psychiatric leaders also maintained that their discipline possessed the knowledge and techniques to identify the appropriate social and environmental changes that presumably optimized mental as well as physical health. Drawing upon wartime experiences, Roy R. Grinker and John P. Speigel insisted that the treatment of individuals—preferably in a noninstitutional setting—had to be accompanied by a program to deal with "the regressive trends within society" (Grinker and Speigel, 1945). Mental hygiene, claimed Robert H. Felix, the first Director of the National Institute of Mental Health (NIMH), and R. V. Bowers in 1948, had to be concerned "with more than the psychoses and with more than hospitalized mental illness." Personality, after all, was shaped by socio-environmental influences. Psychiatry, in collaboration with the social sciences, had to emphasize the problems of the "ambulatory ill and the preambulatory ill (those whose probability of breakdown was high)" (Felix and Bowers, 1948). The community, therefore, was psychiatry's natural habitat, and the specialty had to play a vital role in creating a presumably healthier social order. Indeed, as early as 1945 Felix argued that psychiatry had an obligation to "go out and find the people who need help—and that means, in their local communities" (Felix, 1945). If potential schizophrenics could be identified before the onset of the acute stage, treatment in a community setting might preclude subsequent institutionalization.

Federal Policy Changes and the Postwar Years

The shift in psychiatric theory and the experiences of World War II could hardly by themselves promote major policy and structural innovations. By 1945, however, many of the other structural and intellectual impediments to change had weakened or disappeared. The New Deal had altered in fundamental ways the scope of federal activities and strengthened as well the importance of scientists and intellectuals in the formulation and implementation of policy. World War II not only confirmed these trends but also weakened hereditarian patterns of thought, which were associated with the horrors of Nazism. Environmental ideologies conducive to social activism thus gained in popularity. In the immediate postwar years, the stage was set for a fundamental policy shift that involved basic transformations in the specialty of psychiatry and other mental health professions as well as a new role for the federal government.

Before substantive policy alternatives could even be considered, psychiatrists had to create a more effective organizational vehicle to promote the case for change. In 1945 the structure of psychiatry had changed little since the midnineteenth century. The APA had only two functions:

to hold an annual convention and to publish the *American Journal of Psychiatry*. The association lacked an adequate full-time staff or a secure financial base, and elected officers rarely devoted much time to its affairs. Accountability was thus diffused and the organization never developed systematic or coherent policies.

Between 1945 and 1950 a bitter conflict took place within the APA over the future direction of American psychiatry. In the end, those who sought a wider role for their specialty triumphed. They succeeded in establishing a permanent organizational structure that facilitated the emergence of an activist psychiatry involved with broad individual and social problems. The new focus meant that the APA was no longer preoccupied with public mental hospitals.

The changes in the APA corresponded to an equally profound shift in the location and outlook of members. By 1956 only about 17 percent of the nearly 10,000 members were employed in state hospitals or Veterans Administration facilities. The remainder were either in private practice or working in government or educational agencies, community clinics, or medical schools. This change reflected the dominance of psychodynamic and psychoanalytic psychiatry.

The internal reorganization of American psychiatry was only a precondition for radical changes in public policy; alone the specialty had neither the stature nor the means to influence the public at large or their elected representatives. Before the foundations of a new policy could be laid, therefore, some other means had to be found to promote desirable changes. One alternative was to create a coalition to persuade state legislatures and governors of the necessity for new policy initiatives. In individual states, such a strategy proved successful. Karl and William Menninger, for example, played forceful and decisive roles in Kansas because of their personalities and national visibility. But Kansas was not the nation. Generally speaking, the sheer number and diversity of states posed insuperable obstacles to efforts directed toward policy innovations.

Another alternative was to expand the role of the federal government and create some form of state-federal partnership. The prospects of such a development were not especially bright: Responsibility for care and treatment of the mentally ill still resided with the states. A presidential veto of a land-grant bill in 1854 had ensured that the federal government would play no role in mental health policy. The U.S. Public Health Service's Division of Mental Hygiene, created in 1930, dealt only with narcotic addiction problems. But the enactment of the National Mental Health Act of 1946 ended the tradition of federal inactivity and provided psychiatric activists with an unprecedented opportunity.

In the late 1930s Lawrence C. Kolb, a psychiatrist who headed the Division of Mental Hygiene, undertook a quiet campaign to persuade Congress to establish a National Neuropsychiatric Institute in the Public

Health Service modeled somewhat after the National Cancer Institute. Preoccupation with war-related issues, however, precluded congressional action.

Toward the end of the war, Robert H. Felix, Kolb's successor, revived the proposal but in considerably expanded form. He drafted a bill and enlisted the aid of Congressman J. Percy Priest, who held public hearings in 1945. Shortly thereafter Claude Pepper of Florida, a New Deal Democrat, followed suit in the Senate. The purpose of these hearings was not to investigate the subject of mental illnesses but rather to mobilize support for the idea that the federal government could be a significant participant in mental health policy. At that very same time, a broad coalition of medical and social activists was on the verge of succeeding in their efforts to transform the role of the federal government in health policy by securing legislation (such as the Hill-Burton Act of 1946) that appropriated large subsidies for hospital construction, research, and medical education.

The hearings in both houses revealed that the pressure to act was generated by three groups: a small number of federal officials; concerned laypersons; and a group of psychiatrists whose wartime experiences had reinforced their belief that their specialty had to change. There was little evidence of any groundswell of public support for the measure. Significant opposition, on the other hand, was also absent. Perhaps because the initial level of funding was relatively small, the bill easily passed and became law on July 3, 1946.

The National Mental Health Act had three basic goals: first, to support research relating to the cause, diagnosis, and treatment of neuropsychiatric disorders; second, to train professional personnel in psychiatry by awarding individual fellowships and institutional grants; and, finally, to make grants to states to assist in the establishment of clinics and treatment centers, and to fund demonstration studies dealing with the prevention, diagnosis, and treatment of neuropsychiatric disorders. Financial support for institutional care and treatment of the mentally ill was specifically excluded.

What was most significant about the act was not its specific provisions but rather its general goals and the way in which they were to be implemented. The legislation provided financial and institutional support for research, much of it based on the assumption that the roots of mental illness could be traced to broad social and environmental determinants. Thus, it promoted a social model of mental diseases and an emphasis on community rather than institutional treatment.

Felix's views were suggestive of the shape that mental health ideology and policy would take in subsequent years. In his eyes, mental disorder was "a true public health problem" (Felix, 1946), the resolution of which required more knowledge about the etiology and nature of mental diseases, more effective methods of prevention and treatment, and better trained staff. Although conceding that the mental hospital would be required for the foreseeable future, he insisted that the greatest need was for a large number of outpatient community clinics (probably modeled after prewar child guidance clinics) to serve individuals in the early stages of any mental disease. Not only would these clinics avoid the stigmatization associated with mental hospitals but they would also point the way to effective preventive programs.

In 1949, the National Institute of Mental Health (NIMH) came into formal existence under the provisions of the National Mental Health Act. With the support of NIMH's Community Services Branch, which provided matching federal funds, community mental health programs expanded rapidly. Before 1940 community clinics existed largely to serve the needs of children and delinquents; after 1945 their clientele began to include an adult population. Although hospitals continued to account for the lion's share of state mental health budgets, the presumption was that an alternative community program based on prevention and early treatment would eventually diminish or eliminate the need for hospitalization by identifying pathology in its early stages. "The guiding philosophy which permeates the activities of the National Institute of Mental Health." Felix told his APA colleagues in 1949, "is that prevention of mental illness, and the production of positive mental health, is an attainable goal" (Felix, 1949).

In the immediate postwar era, a series of spectacular exposés (visual as well as verbal) by such journalists as Albert Deutsch, Albert Q. Maisel, Frank L. Wright, and Mike Gorman, as well as the publication of Mary Jane Ward's best-selling novel *The Snake Pit,* riveted public attention on psychiatry as well as scandalous conditions in state mental hospitals. The decline in the image and quality of institutional care heightened the attractiveness of alternative approaches.

Changes in State Policy

Slowly but surely the developments of the immediate postwar years began to influence state policy. In 1949 the Governors' Conference commenced an active role in seeking new ways of dealing with mental health problems. It sponsored a wide-ranging study of mental health programs, which was completed the following year. Although concerned with the necessity of improving conditions in state mental hospitals, the report also called for other kinds of services, "since clinical and community care" was "much more economical than institutional treatment." Indeed, it recommended that outpatient clinics provide assistance "for persons in need of help, but not of hospitalization" and called for the establishment of programs "which look toward prevention and the maintenance and strengthening of mental health" (Council of State Governments, 1950). In 1954 a special Governors' Conference on Mental Health adopted a program urging expansion of efforts in the areas of community services, treatment, rehabilitation, and aftercare. During the 1950s state policy tended to pursue two goals that were not, at least at that time, inherently contradictory: improvement of institutional care and expansion of community services.

The growing emphasis on community programs was given considerable support by the Milbank Memorial Fund—an influential and respected philanthropic foundation long involved in health issues. During the 1950s the annual conferences of the Milbank Fund emphasized a social and environmental etiology and devoted considerable attention to the planning and evaluation of the activities of a number of community mental health projects. Psychiatrists traditionally had insisted on the removal of patients from an inappropriate environment and their placement in a structured and controlled one (that is, the mental hospital) where the mind could be redirected and the disease process reversed. The emphasis on community care and treatment represented a profound shift in psychiatric thinking. Admittedly, the conferences never concluded that state mental hospitals were obsolete (although they were cognizant of the fact that, in a state such as New York, about one-third of its total budget was allocated to mental health, making this item an obvious target to those with different priorities). On the contrary, participants assumed a continuum of care from hospitalization (either in general or mental hospitals) to outpatient facilities. Those involved also accepted as an article of faith (but with little persuasive evidence) that the population at risk could be identified and that early detection and treatment were the key to programmatic success and to a more effective use of fiscal resources.

All too often the rhetoric of community care and treatment so prevalent in the immediate postwar years is ignored. Yet rhetoric cannot be dismissed so easily. Rhetoric, after all, shapes agendas and debates; it creates expectations that in turn mold policies; and it informs socialization, training, and education of those in professional occupations. During the 1950s, for example, the rhetoric of the advocates of community care and treatment led many states to experiment with new policy initiatives. New York and California led the way. In 1954 the former enacted the famous and influential Community Mental Health Services Act. Under its provisions any county or city could create a local mental health board, which was empowered to subsidize four kinds of services: outpatient psychiatric clinics; inpatient psychiatric services in general hospitals; psychiatric rehabilitation services; and consultant and educational services. The state in turn would reimburse the community for up to one-half of its costs up to a maximum of $1 per capita per year. Two years after passage of this legislation, twenty-one local governments representing nearly 85 percent of the state's population were participating in the program. By 1961 the progam covered 159 outpatient clinics, 21 general hospitals (with 2,194 beds), and 7 rehabilitation services, as well as consultation and educational services. In California the passage of the Short-Doyle Act (or Community Mental Health Services Act) also promoted the growth of local mental health services by using matching state funds.

The Work of the Joint Commission on Mental Illness and Health

New York and California were by no means alone in seeking to redefine, at least in part, the traditional state reliance on hospitalization. Other states followed their examples. The expansion of community facilities was accompanied by new services to schools, courts, and social agencies by nonmedical mental health professionals—a development that offered dramatic evidence of the degree to which the public accepted the importance of psychological services in noninstitutional settings. Nevertheless, state-by-state campaigns for expanded community services posed some difficulties. This was because the influence of psychiatrists tended to be concentrated in a relatively small number of jurisdictions.

Given the experiences of the New Deal, World War II, and the growing role of the federal government in health-related matters in the postwar era, many felt that the time was ripe for another policy departure that would shift part of the burden from the states to the national government. The passage of the National Mental Health Act in 1946 was but a beginning; what was required was legislation that provided for direct federal subsidies for mental health services. A biomedical lobby was now in existence and flourishing, and new policy initiatives were likely to receive a sympathetic reception in Congress. Equally significant, a national campaign could employ the media to bring a message of hope to an eager and enthusiastic public trustful of the claims of mental health experts from both the medical profession as well as from the social sciences. The growing significance of social science in the postwar era undoubtedly added legitimacy to the clamor for change.

To expand the role of the federal government in mental health required strategic planning. In 1953, Dr. Kenneth Appel, then president of the APA, proposed that "a sociological study of the breakdown crisis in the administration of state mental hospital functions" be undertaken (Appel, 1953). He secured the active support of the APA and the American Medical Association (AMA), and in January 1955, these organizations created a Joint Commission on Mental Illness and Health. This commission was to prepare a survey and recommend a national program to improve methods and facilities for the diagnosis, treatment, and care of the mentally ill and mentally retarded, as well as for the promotion of mental health. Other professional and academic organizations quickly added their endorsement. At the same time, a drive was launched to secure the approval (and financial support) of the federal government. With bipartisan support, the Mental Health Study Act became law in July 1955. Under its provisions, Congress endorsed a broad nongovernmental investigation of the "human and economic problems of mental illness" and authorized the Public Health Service to provide grants for the survey (*U.S. Statutes*, 1955). The stage was now set for the Joint Commission on Mental Illness and Health (JCMIH) to begin its work.

Beneath the consensus regarding the need for a national policy lay some unresolved issues. The debate between competing models of health and disease, for example, was by no means resolved. Was the JCMIH to focus on the mentally ill or mental health? Dr. Jack Ewalt (staff director of the JCMIH) and his coworkers adopted a twofold objective: first, to amass data that shed light on the prevalance, diagnosis, treatment, care, and rehabilitation of mental disorders; and second, to use this data as the basis for a "radical reconceptualization of the problems and possibly a reconstruction of the institutions so that resource use might be more economical and mental health better served" (Ewalt, 1956). Significantly, the commission's staff included individuals from the social and behavioral sciences as well as psychiatry.

The joint commission's final report, *Action for Mental Health*, was released to the public in March 1961. Its analyses and recommendations were broad rather than technical or narrow, and in many respects they mirrored much of the thinking of the postwar years. The document embodied a psychosocial and psychodynamic approach; it stressed the necessity for environmental approaches to the problems of mental health within integrated community settings. The report emphasized the rejection of the mentally ill; Americans remained uncomfortable with the mentally ill—as they were not with the physically ill—despite their broad sympathies and good intentions toward the former. *Action for Mental Health* argued for a diversified program: a much larger investment in basic research; a partnership between psychiatry and nonmedical mental health workers (but with due attention to their respective competencies); a national recruitment and training program for those involved in providing services; a greater effort to make services available to "mentally troubled individuals" in order to forestall more serious breakdowns; intensive treatment of the acute mentally ill in community mental health clinics, general hospitals, and mental hospitals; provision for aftercare, intermediate care, and rehabilitation services for released patients; and a bold attempt to educate the American public to recognize mental illnesses and to support a national program. The report further demanded that no state hospitals of more than a thousand beds be built; that no patients be admitted to any existing facility having more than a thousand beds; and that all state hospitals be converted "into centers for the long-term and combined care of chronic diseases, including mental illness." Its fiscal recommendations were equally remarkable: Members asked that expenditures for public mental patient services be doubled in the next five years and tripled in the next ten, and urged an expansion in the fiscal role of the federal government well beyond a commitment to research and training (Joint Commission, 1961).

The reception of *Action for Mental Health,* though generally favorable, was by no means one-sided. Indeed, it would have been surprising if the report's recommendations had been received without controversy. Some psychiatrists were concerned that the legitimacy of their specialty might be affected adversely by a shift of many functions to other non-medical mental health professionals; some disliked the concept of inclusive chronic hospitals; some rejected the proposition that psychiatric illnesses were almost entirely of psychological origin and insisted that biological factors were involved; some felt that a limitation on the size of mental hospitals was "premature," if only because size and quality were not necessarily related; and others expressed the view that the report was far too sweeping and vague.

Opposition to the work of the joint commission also came from individuals who had been long associated with state mental hospitals, many of whom were resentful about the actual and implied criticisms. Moreover, during the 1950s, an interdisciplinary group of psychiatrists and social scientists had developed the concept of the therapeutic community, which was based on the assumption that it was possible to create institutional environments conducive to therapeutic and humane goals. To this group, the problem was not institutions per se but rather the manner in which they were organized, structured, and administered, and the goal, in creating therapeutic communities, was the reform—not the abolition—of institutional care.

Action for Mental Health was a broad and inclusive document that spelled out a vision for the future rather than a specific legislative program. Moreover, the complexities of a decentralized political system precluded the adoption of a unified program. Those who were concerned with the mentally ill, therefore, were faced with the task of drawing up some kind of legislative agenda capable of attracting broad support. Given the traditional role of the states in mental health policy, it was not surprising that state officials took part in a broad-based coalition to promote the passage of federal legislation that would open up new sources of funding.

In November 1961, a Special Governors' Conference in Mental Health was convened to consider the recommendations of the JCMIH. The policy statement finally adopted by the conference reflected the thinking of that period: a preference for community-based treatment, with cost sharing by localities and states; the further development of psychiatric services in general hospitals; an expansion of research and training; an emphasis on the use of counseling skills of such groups as teachers, clergy, and law enforcement officials; the unification and integration of state mental health activities; and a cost-sharing policy involving federal, state, and local governments. The cost-sharing recommendation was probably of paramount concern to state officials, given the large expenditures associated with existing mental hospital systems. The conference arranged for representatives of the Advisory Commission on Intergovernmental Relations to contact the White House in order to draft appropriate legislation.

The Development of a New Federal Policy

By 1961 public sentiment appeared to be supportive of new mental health policy initiatives. Concern for the mentally ill for much of American history had been generally confined to families with members who demonstrated aberrant behavior that seemed threatening; in the postwar era, however, psychological interventions—notably psychotherapy—to deal with personal problems had become increasingly popular. The continuum model that blurred the distinction between mental health and mental disease was now accepted by a wide public. Thus, all of the elements for a new policy seemed favorable; the remaining task was to tap the massive financial resources of the federal government.

That those committed to new policies turned to the federal government was not surprising. During the 1960s social activists manifested little confidence in state policy making; they had far greater faith in the ability of the federal government to develop new priorities and programs and to provide adequate levels of funding. The prevailing consensus of that decade was that states had failed to meet their social welfare responsibilities. Hence, many activists, even though paying homage to the concept of a federal-state partnership, promoted policies that tended to diminish the role or authority of state governments. They received indirect support from NIMH officials, who tended to identify state governments with an obsolete emphasis on institutional care.

The election of John F. Kennedy in 1960 augured well for the hopes of those dedicated to an expanded federal role in mental health policy. Unlike his predecessor, Kennedy seemed favorably disposed, although his basic concern was with mental retardation rather than the mental illnesses. In late 1961 Kennedy asked Abraham Ribicoff, secretary of the Department of Health, Education and Welfare (HEW), to examine the report of the JCMIH in order to develop an appropriate federal policy. Ribicoff was specifically instructed to deal with the issue of institutional versus noninstitutional services. He set up a presidential interagency committee to develop a coherent program.

28

From the very outset, it was clear that the proponents of a community-oriented program had the upper hand. Felix (and other like-minded individuals in key positions) played a decisive role; his position as director of NIMH enabled him both to set the agenda and to control the information that served as the basis for policy discussions. In collaboration with Stanley Yolles (deputy director at NIMH) and other staff, Felix developed a series of recommendations that made the community mental health center the primary recipient of federal funds. In January 1962, Ribicoff endorsed the view that early diagnosis and treatment in the community would eventually obviate the need for large state mental hospitals.

By the end of 1962, Anthony Celebrezze, Ribicoff's successor at HEW, accepted the recommendations of the task force. "We are of the strong opinion," he informed the White House,

> that the prevention of mental illness is as important as the care and treatment of the severely mentally ill. Moreover, we disagree with the heavy emphasis in the [JCMIH] Report on increasing services to the severely mentally ill within State hospital systems. Rather, we take the position that primary interest in future mental health programs should be improvement of the mental health of the people of the community through a continuum of local services, not just upon the treatment and rehabilitative aspects of these programs. We are especially impressed with the need for local initiative in working out community programs utilizing various public and private agencies. We believe that primary efforts to prevent mental illness must start in childhood and depend on the work of many social institutions—for example, the family, the church, the school, and public and private health and welfare agencies [Celebrezze, 1962].

To achieve these goals, Celebrezze recommended the following measures: planning grants for community mental health programs; funds for the construction of as many as 500 community mental health centers by 1970; special project grants to state mental hospitals to implement demonstration projects aimed at releasing patients to their homes; and funding for research and training. He specifically excluded the use of federal money to relieve states of their responsibilities for financing institutional care.

The story of the development of mental health policy from the recommendations of the task force to the passage of the Mental Retardation Facilities and Community Mental Health Centers Construction Act of 1963 is a lengthy and complex one. Suffice it to say that President John F. Kennedy threw the weight and prestige of his office behind the advocates of a community-oriented program. In his message to Congress in February 1963, he proposed a new and radical national mental health program. "This approach," he stated, "relies primarily upon the new knowledge and new drugs acquired and developed in recent years which make it possible for most of the mentally ill to be successfully and quickly treated in their own communities and returned to a useful place in society." Such "breakthroughs," he added, "have rendered obsolete . . . a prolonged or permanent confinement in huge, unhappy mental hospitals" (Kennedy, 1963).

That the initiative of the Kennedy administration departed in some fundamental ways from the recommendations of the JCMIH was largely either overlooked or ignored. Indeed, Kennedy urged the establishment of *centers:* the joint commission had spoken about *clinics.* Perhaps the difference between the two terms did not appear to be overwhelming, but it is clear that the former was far more inclusive and presumed not the strengthening of an existing policy but rather the creation of a new policy. Indeed, the designation of the new entities as "centers" evoked an image of a physical structure but did not define its functions or its relationship to mental hospitals. In the ensuing testimony before congressional committees (much of which was orchestrated), the rhetoric of the community mental health centers ideology became overpowering. There was little disposition on the part of either Senate or House members to question the foundation on which the new proposal rested. Rhetoric rather than reality carried the day. The rejection of the traditional policy of institutional care and treatment and its replacement by a new departure was formally confirmed when the new act became law in October 1963. The civil rights movement and the development of public interest law during the remainder of the decade carried forward the impetus to diminish the role of mental hospitals in mental health policy.

Consequences of the New Policy

By the early 1960s the foundations of the long-standing tradition of institutional care had been undermined. Indeed, hospital populations declined rapidly after 1965. A shift in thinking had made community care and treatment, at least in theory, an acceptable alternative to institutionalization. Administrative and structural changes within institutions, including open-door policies, informal admissions, and efforts to prepare patients for early release, as well as the introduction of psychotropic drugs, reinforced the belief that treatment could be provided in the community.

One of the most significant factors in the decline in hospital populations was the establishment of Medicaid and Medicare. This legislation stimulated the growth of chronic nursing homes, and many aged persons formerly cared for in mental hospitals were sent to them. State officials were enthusiastic about this development, since this transferred fiscal responsibility for many aged individuals to the federal government. At the same time, the rapid expansion of third-party reimbursement plans stimulated use of inpatient and outpatient psychiatric services in general hospitals.

The enthusiasm of the 1960s, however, could not conceal the fact that a coherent policy had yet to be defined. The reduction of the patient population undoubtedly improved the lives of those remaining in state hospitals. Nevertheless, the consequences of postwar innovations in mental health policy were hardly an unmixed blessing. The federal initiative, oddly enough, diminished the role and authority of states by forging a de facto policy that made the community mental health center—not the state mental hospital—the major component of the mental health system. Yet there was no effort to define the basic functions of such centers or to develop mechanisms to ensure some measure of integration with a state hospital system that, whatever its shortcomings, had traditionally provided minimum levels of care for the mentally ill.

In ensuing years, the mentally ill previously cared for in mental hospitals were thrust into communities that were unable or unwilling to provide supportive care. Ironically, during an era when resources for mental health were growing rapidly and psychiatric and psychological services were expanding to include new categories of individuals, the needs of the severely mentally ill were sometimes overlooked as other priorities took precedence. The continued presence of the severely mentally ill still represents a challenge to the postwar generation's vision that community treatment, prevention, and social activism would resolve, once and for all, the problems posed by mental illness.

Bibliographical Note

The research for this chapter was supported by a grant from the National Institute of Mental Health (MH 39030), Public Health Service, U.S. Department of Health and Human Services. This project will culminate in a book dealing with mental health policy from 1940 to 1970. I have examined a large number of manuscript collections of individuals and organizations, oral history transcripts, state and federal government documents, journals and newspapers, and books. To have provided references for this chapter would have taken an inordinate amount of space; I have therefore only given citations to direct quotations. Examples of the sources used in the preparation of this chapter can be found in my articles, "Psychiatry and Social Activism: The Politics of a Specialty in Postwar America," *Bulletin of the History of Medicine,* 1986, *60* (4), 477-501, and "The Forging of Mental Health Policy in America: World War II to New Frontier," *Journal of the History of Medicine*, 1987, *42* (4).

I have not dealt with the introduction of the psychotropic drugs in 1954, which many assume began the process of "deinstitutionalization." There are several reasons for this omission. First, the final report of the JCMIH noted the use of drugs but pointed out that its effects on the size of hospital populations were modest. Second, its members, while conceding the usefulness of these drugs, were not persuaded that they represented any panacea. (Indeed, there is striking evidence that the psychiatric attitude toward drugs ultimately proved more realistic that the perceptions found in the popular media and general public or the claims of drug companies.) Finally, there is persuasive statistical evidence that the decline in state mental hospital populations immediately following the introduction of drugs about 1955 was relatively modest; the greatest decline occurred after the passage of Medicaid and Medicare legislation.

References

Appel, K. E. "A Program for Public Support." American Psychiatric Association Mental Hospital Institute, *Proceedings*, 1953, *5*, 1–8.
Celebrezze, A. to J. F. Kennedy, November 30, 1962. White House Central Files, Box 338, HE 1-1, John F. Kennedy Library, Boston, Massachusetts.
Council of State Governments. *The Mental Health Programs of the Forty-Eight States: A Report to the Governors' Conference.* Chicago: Council of State Governments, 1950.
Ewalt, J. R. "Evaluating Mental Health Programs." Presentation at National Opinion Research Center, August 9, 1956, Chicago, Illinois. Joint Commission on Mental Illness and Health Papers, Box 2, American Psychiatric Association Archives, Washington, D.C.
Felix, R. H. "Mental Public Health: A Blueprint." Presentation at St. Elizabeth Hospital, Washington, D.C., April 21, 1945. R. H. Felix Papers, Box 1, National Library of Medicine, Bethesda, Maryland.
Felix, R. H. "Developing a Federal Mental Health Program." National Conference of Social Work, *Proceedings*, 1946, *73*, 447–455.
Felix, R. H. "Mental Disorders as a Public Health Problem." *American Journal of Psychiatry*, 1949, *106*, 401–406.
Felix, R. H., and Bowers, R. V. "Mental Hygiene and Socio-Environmental Factors." *Milbank Memorial Fund Quarterly*, 1948, *26*, 125–147.
Grinker, R. R., and Spiegel, J. P. *Men Under Stress.* Philadelphia: Blakiston, 1945.
Joint Commission on Mental Illness and Health. *Action for Mental Health: Final Report of the Joint Commission on Mental Illness and Health.* New York: Basic Books, 1961.
Kennedy, J. F. "Mental Illness and Mental Retardation: Message from the President of the United States." 88th Congress, First Session, *House Document No. 58* (February 5, 1963).
Menninger, W. C. "Psychiatric Experience in the War, 1941–1946." *American Journal of Psychiatry*, 1946, *103*, 577–586.
U.S. Statutes at Large, Chapter 417, 1955, *69*, 381–383.

Gerald N. Grob is professor of history and member of the Institute for Health, Health Care Policy, and Aging Research, Rutgers University.

Help-seeking research indicates that a number of cultural, social, and organizational factors trigger or inhibit contact with mental health professionals. The impact of each of these factors has changed considerably in recent years.

Help-Seeking Processes and Mental Health Services

Allan V. Horwitz

Help-seeking behaviors form the critical link between the emergence of psychiatric illnesses, on one hand, and the provision of mental health services, on the other. The initial recognition that someone needs help usually occurs in the lay community. People define psychiatric symptoms in varying ways and use many alternatives to mental health systems in response to troubling conditions. The organization and accessibility of treatment services also influence help seeking. The interactions among psychiatric conditions, social and cultural predispositions to seek treatment, and the organization of mental health services are the central concerns of help-seeking studies. The goal of these studies is to specify the factors that lead some people to enter the mental health system and some to deal with comparable conditions in other ways.

In some contexts, people readily consider themselves in need of psychiatric help and view mental health professionals as valued resources (Kadushin, 1969). Most individuals, however, are not likely to define themselves or others as needing psychiatric help but instead interpret symptoms as personality flaws, somatic difficulties, or transitory phenomena (Clausen and Yarrow, 1955). Their reluctance to interpret problems as signs of mental illness often leads them to seek help from general medical providers, clergy, spiritualists, or a host of other practitioners

D. Mechanic (ed.). *Improving Mental Health Services: What the Social Sciences Can Tell Us.*
New Directions for Mental Health Services, no. 36. San Francisco: Jossey-Bass, 1987.

outside the mental health system. Others seek no help at all and enter psychiatric treatment when families or community members mobilize the police to deal with their bizarre and disruptive behaviors. The predisposing factors that may propel people into or may restrain them from entering mental health systems include cultural orientations, material resources, and social support.

Predisposing conditions are themselves shaped by the organization of the mental health system. The availability, structure, and type of mental health services, the characteristics of psychiatric professionals, and the system of financial reimbursement for psychiatric treatment all influence the extent and nature of help-seeking efforts. Together, these organizational influences and predisposing conditions shape selection processes. The challenge for help-seeking research is to discern whether mental health services adequately provide care for people who need them or whether there could be a better match between client need and service provision.

The Prevalence of Help-Seeking Behavior

A notable finding of population surveys is that only a minority of persons with diagnosable psychiatric conditions seek help from mental health professionals. For example, in the comprehensive Epidemiological Catchment Area (ECA) studies, data from New Haven, Baltimore, and St. Louis show that, during the six-month period prior to the interview, only between 8.1 and 12.4 percent of individuals with a recent diagnosis reported a contact in the mental health specialty sector (Shapiro and others, 1984). In no diagnostic category did a majority of people with a recent disorder seek care for a mental health reason during the prior six-month period. The highest proportion of cases currently in treatment across the three sites reached 48.1 percent for schizophrenia. On the other hand, help seeking from mental health professionals was especially low for persons with cognitive or substance abuse disorders.

Research on the lifetime prevalence of treated and untreated psychiatric disorders indicates that most people with clinical conditions never enter mental health treatment systems. A comprehensive review that measured both the prevalence of mental disorder in population samples and the extent of contact with mental health professionals in eleven studies conducted between 1917 and 1973 found that a median 26.7 percent of diagnosed cases of psychopathology had ever entered treatment (Link and Dohrenwend, 1980). The seven studies that examined psychotic disorders reported that 59.7 percent of diagnosed cases of all psychosis and 83.3 percent of schizophrenic cases underwent treatment at some point. The majority of people with clinically significant disorders and sizable proportions with severe problems receive no treatment from mental health professionals.

Because only a minority of psychiatrically impaired individuals seek help from mental health professionals does not mean that others receive no treatment whatever for their disorders. Indeed, most people with psychiatric disorders consult medical doctors about their problems (Goldberg and Huxley, 1980). Many psychiatric disorders encompass somatic as well as psychological symptoms, and patients naturally may focus on the physical component of their complaints. In addition, the presentation of somatic rather than psychiatric complaints provides a more comfortable and less stigmatizing way of obtaining help for emotional problems (Balint, 1957).

Community surveys indicate that nearly half of respondents with diagnosed psychiatric disorders who seek some professional treatment utilize the general medical, rather than the psychiatric specialty, sector for help (Leaf and others, 1985). These patients include many severely ill individuals as well as people with relatively minor symptoms. Conversely, a significant proportion of patients in primary-care settings primarily suffer from psychiatric rather than somatic difficulties (Tessler, Mechanic, and Dimond, 1976; Anderson, Francis, Lion, and Daughety, 1977). Moreover, the majority of patients with psychiatric problems who are treated by primary-care physicians do not seek further help in the specialty mental health sector (Goldberg and Huxley, 1980).

Little systematic data exists on the extent to which people use alternatives to the psychiatric or general medical sectors for mental health problems. Many people seek help from a range of providers including clergy, spiritualists, or self-help groups, while others utilize intimates or make no help-seeking efforts whatever (Garrison, 1977; Horwitz, 1977b). Who these people are, what targets of help seeking they use, and what effects result remain important questions for further investigation.

Despite the fact that a majority of persons with clinically significant disorders do not enter the mental health sector, help seeking from mental health professionals has increased dramatically in recent years. The organization of mental health services is now far more conducive to voluntary help seeking than in the past. Beginning in the 1960s, the development of community mental health centers, the growth of outpatient facilities in communities and general hospitals, the improvement of benefits for psychiatric care provided by private and nonprofit insurance programs, and the expansion of public programs such as Medicaid that help fund mental health services for the poor led to a vast expansion of outpatient psychiatric services (Mechanic, 1980). Community mental health centers and outpatient facilities are now the largest source of treatment in the mental health specialty sector, having increased from 379,000 clinical episodes in 1955 to 4,600,000 episodes in 1975 to 7,000,000 in 1985 (Kramer, 1977; National Institute of Mental Health, 1987).

Population surveys also indicate a growing readiness to utilize psychiatric services. In one large national survey conducted in 1957 and again in 1976, the number of people who would use professional help to deal with personal problems rose from one-third to one-half and the number who actually used help nearly doubled (Veroff, Kulka, and Douvan, 1981). Indeed, in the 1976 interviews, 26 percent of adults had sought professional help for personal problems.

The growing restrictiveness of inpatient facilities servicing the severely mentally ill contrasts with the expansion of outpatient services for the less seriously disturbed. The nature of severe psychiatric illnesses often prevents persons with these disorders from seeking help voluntarily. Instead, families and community members typically initiate psychiatric help seeking. In the past, these people could direct their help-seeking efforts toward inpatient institutions and successfully commit disturbed members (Scheff, 1964). Since the late 1960s, however, the rights of potential mental patients have greatly expanded as legislation and court orders have established narrow criteria for involuntary commitments, expanded procedural rights for persons facing commitment, and increased involvement of lawyers in commitment proceedings (Gove, Tovo, and Hughes, 1985). Over the past thirty years, commitment rates have declined considerably for all population groups except minor children (Lerman, 1982; Taube and Barrett, 1985).

These changes mean that help seeking for severe mental illness now occurs in a radically different context than previously. Families can no longer take for granted that institutions are available to take responsibility for disordered relatives (Morrissey, Tessler, and Farrin, 1979). Yet the mental health system has not found effective ways of bringing chronically mentally ill people into treatment in the absence of involuntary commitment mechanisms. The result has been an increased caretaking burden on the families of the severely mentally ill, a growth in advocacy organizations promoting the interests of families, and heightened tensions between families and professionals (Tessler, Killian, and Gubman, 1987).

Predisposing Factors in Help-Seeking Behavior

Many factors account for why some disordered individuals enter psychiatric treatment, some seek alternative sources of help, and others resist any assistance. Sociologists have been especially interested in how different cultural definitions of personal problems, attitudes toward mental health professionals, and the availability of social support in the community facilitate or impede help seeking from professionals. Here, I briefly examine how these factors vary across divergent social class, gender, age, and relational statuses.

Social Class. A consistent finding of epidemiological surveys is that rates of mental illness vary inversely with socioeconomic status (Link and Dohrenwend, 1980; Robins and others, 1984). On the other hand, rates of treated mental illness vary directly with social class. Higher status groups whose cultural orientations are most congruent with the introspective and psychological norms of the mental health professions have the greatest propensity toward psychiatric help seeking. In contrast, members of socioeconomic groups rarely initiate psychiatric help seeking but enter mental health systems through referrals from physicians, social agencies, or agents of social control (Hollingshead and Redlich, 1958; Goldberg and Huxley, 1980).

Studies in the 1950s and 1960s found highly distinct patterns in psychiatric help seeking among the social classes (Hollingshead and Redlich, 1958; Myers and Roberts, 1959; Lowenthal, 1964; Kadushin, 1969). Members of different classes varied widely in the extent to which they attributed problems to psychiatric causes. Upper-class people were likely to define and seek help for a wide range of emotional and interpersonal disturbances. They sought treatment near the emergence of the first signs of disorder through self-referrals or referrals from family or friends. Similarly, ethnic groups such as Jews who are marked by high levels of introspection, cosmopolitan orientations, and participation in reference groups supportive of psychotherapy are highly represented in outpatient therapies (Srole and others, 1962). Indeed, in one large national sample, over 50 percent of Jewish respondents had utilized professional help for psychiatric problems—a percentage far higher than that of other ethnic groups (Veroff, Kulka, and Douvan, 1981).

In contrast, lower-class persons are likely to interpret mental problems as symptomatic of physical problems or negative personality traits such as laziness or drunkenness. Their problems commonly come to the attention of the mental health system when they display aggressive or bizarre behavior. The police, courts, social agencies, and clinics usually initiate referrals into treatment for lower-class people. Different ethnic groups illustrate similar patterns. Members of ethnic groups such as Chinese or Hispanics who have little congruence with psychiatric culture resist help seeking from mental health professionals (Garrison, 1977; Lin, Tardiff, Donetz, and Goresky, 1978).

Studies that separate the components of social class differences generally find that education is more important than income in accounting for help seeking (Gurin, Veroff, and Field, 1960; Veroff, Kulka, and Douvan, 1981). In particular, participation in liberal and humanistic culture facilitates contact with mental health professionals. Kadushin (1969), for example, found that the primary clients of outpatient psychiatric care in New York City went to plays, concerts, museums, and art galleries, and worked in occupations that stress the artistic and psychological, such as the health professions, teaching, the arts, and communications. Clients of private psychiatrists similarly are far more likely than their proportion in the population to be drawn from the humanistic professions (Marmor, 1975). Studies of college students also show that psychiatric help seeking is particularly prevalent among humanities and social science majors (especially psychology), viewers of foreign films, and holders of "cosmopolitan" value systems (Greenley and Mechanic, 1976).

In the past, these cultural differences resulted in highly divergent rates of treatment across social classes. For example, in a large community study of individuals in midtown Manhattan in the early 1950s, among people who were rated as psychiatrically impaired, more than twice as many upper-class persons as members of other social classes had received psychiatric treatment at some time (Srole and others, 1962). More recent research, however, shows a dramatic narrowing in the use of psychiatric services across social classes. There now are minimal class and ethnic differences in the proportion of diagnosed psychiatric cases utilizing outpatient psychiatric services, although the extent of class differences in the pathways into treatment is unknown (Tischler, Henisz, Myers, and Boswell, 1975; Stern, 1977; Veroff, Kulka, and Douvan, 1981; Leaf and others, 1987).

Several factors account for the changing relationship between social class and psychiatric help seeking. Access to and awareness of psychiatric resources has expanded, and facilities are now more likely to be present in low-income and minority areas of major cities. In addition, the growth of third-party and public reimbursement has minimized cost differentials that presented resource barriers to psychiatric care in the past. The expansion of social service agencies has also led lower-income persons to be in contact with more professionals who make referrals to mental health services. Finally, a concern with psychological adjustment and attitudes favorable to psychiatry may be more broadly distributed across American culture than previously (Veroff, Kulka, and Douvan, 1981). The result has been to transform psychiatric help seeking from the concern of a small, psychiatrically sophisticated elite group to a process utilized by many segments of the population.

Gender. There are no consistent gender differences in overall rates of treatment from mental health providers among people who have been identified as psychiatrically disordered in community studies (Link and Dohrenwend, 1980; Fox, 1984; Leaf and Bruce, 1987). Yet substantial differences exist in how men and women react to psychiatric symptoms and seek help for them. Women show greater readiness to define their problems in psychiatric terms, while men resist admitting personal vulnerabilities (Veroff, Kulka, and Douvan, 1981). Given the perception of a psychiatric problem, women more readily think of themselves as in need of help and discuss their difficulties with other people (Horwitz, 1977a;

Kessler, Brown, and Broman, 1981). Women also predominate among those who seek help for mental health problems from primary-care physicians (Leaf and Bruce, 1987). Finally, women are more likely to use outpatient services, while men predominate in inpatient facilities (Tudor, Tudor, and Gove, 1977; Taube and Barrett, 1985).

Women not only initiate help seeking more often for themselves but also play a more active part in psychiatric help seeking for intimates. Wives are more prone than husbands to recognize the psychiatric problems of spouses, respond sympathetically and provide support to them, and participate actively in the help-seeking process (Horwitz, 1977a; Clausen, Pfeffer, and Huffine, 1982; Ginsberg and Brown, 1982). In one recent study, wives were twice as likely to play a major role in their husband's reentry into treatment than were husbands of female patients (Clausen, Pfeffer, and Huffine, 1982).

Gender differences in help seeking stem from sex-linked cultural expectations and socialization experiences regarding appropriate responses to emotional problems. Yet the readiness of women and reluctance of men to interpret their problems in psychological frameworks and seek psychiatric help may have been more distinct in the past than at present. The ways in which the sexes respond to psychiatric problems seem to be converging, particularly as men become less resistant to using mental health services (Fox, 1984; Leaf and Bruce, 1987).

Age. Epidemiological research shows no constant relationship between age and the overall prevalence of mental disorder (Link and Dohrenwend, 1980; Robins and others, 1984). On the other hand, age is one of the strongest correlates of psychiatric help seeking. A consistent finding in community surveys is that the proportion of disturbed people who seek psychiatric treatment peaks among twenty-five- to forty-four-year-olds and then declines sharply (Link and Dohrenwend, 1980; Veroff, Kulka, and Douvan, 1981; Fox, 1984; George and others, 1987). In contrast, people over sixty-five are the most likely age group to seek help for psychiatric problems from general medical providers (George and others, 1987).

The reluctance of the elderly to seek help within the mental health system may stem from their socialization in a period when psychiatric help was stigmatized as being associated with madness. They are most comfortable interpreting their problems in somatic frameworks and seeking care from their physicians. Younger groups, however, have been socialized in an era of mental health promotion to view mental health professionals as appropriate help providers. If this interpretation is correct, longitudinal studies of help seeking in future decades will not find the same declining use of psychiatric services with advancing age that typifies current research. Alternatively, the tendency of the elderly to somatize psychiatric problems may have more to do with the greater prevalence of physical disorders at older ages than with cultural and socialization experiences (Cleary, 1986).

Younger persons who are severely mentally ill deviate from the above pattern. They have not been socialized to years of institutional residence and make different kinds of demands on service systems than previous patients (Bachrach, Talbott, and Meyerson, 1987). Earlier generations of seriously ill patients were often compliant and accepted psychiatric services. Contemporary young chronic patients, in contrast, often do not define themselves as mentally ill and commonly express hostile and rejecting attitudes toward mental health professionals (Pepper and Ryglewicz, 1982).

The help-seeking patterns of this group are marked by frequent appearances in the emergency rooms of general hospitals after drug overdoses, suicide attempts, or psychotic episodes followed by short stays in inpatient facilities (Schwartz and Goldfinger, 1981). Police are common referral agents into treatment, following aggressive or self-destructive episodes. Other young chronically mentally ill remain in the community resisting attempts at psychiatric intervention yet lacking informal networks of social support (Segal, Baumohl, and Johnson, 1977). Their hostility toward psychiatry coupled with their isolation from traditional family and community sources of social support present a severe barrier to help seeking among many younger severely mentally ill people. Whether this population will become more amenable to treatment in the mental health system as they age or maintain their antagonistic attitudes is an open question.

Social Relationships. The patterns of relationships between people as well as cultural attitudes and beliefs influence help-seeking patterns. Among those who are identified as psychiatric cases, socially isolated people have more contacts with both the general medical sector (Goldberg and Huxley, 1980) and the mental health specialty sector (Link and Dohrenwend, 1980; Fox, 1984; Leaf and others, 1987). For example, married people are more embedded than unmarried ones in social support networks. Studies consistently show low rates of help seeking among the married and high rates among those who are not currently married, although in some cases help seeking is most prominent among the divorced (Fox, 1984) and in others among the never married (Link and Dohrenwend, 1980). Other groups who lack social support, such as the unemployed, those who live alone, and those with no religion, also utilize medical and mental health services for personal problems more often than those with social support (Goldberg and Huxley, 1980).

The presence of strong relational networks often impedes seeking professional help. People with large and stable relational networks receive more informal support, remain in the community for longer periods of time, and enter hospitals with more severe disorders than those with weaker networks (Lowenthal, 1964; Gillis and Keet, 1965; Horwitz, 1977b). This may in part explain why members of ethnic groups marked by extended familial networks such as Chinese or Mexicans are low utilizers of mental health services. In contrast, isolation from social support networks often leads to quicker use of psychiatric services. Seeking help from professionals may be one way that isolated people obtain support in modern societies.

Relational and cultural factors together influence help-seeking processes (Friedson, 1970). When dense networks with high support also maintain favorable attitudes toward psychiatry, help seeking may be facilitated. For example, individuals with strong support networks in settings such as cosmopolitan metropolitan areas or university towns readily seek help from mental health professionals (Kadushin, 1969). Conversely, isolated individuals who are hostile toward or ignorant of psychiatric culture are highly unlikely to seek professional help. This is the case among the young chronic population who typically lack both family and community support yet reject mental health services (Pepper and Ryglewicz, 1982). While the weakness of social ties usually facilitates help seeking, in some cases social isolation impedes these efforts.

Conclusions

Social, cultural, and organizational changes have led to a great expansion of help seeking from mental health professionals in recent years. Rates of voluntary help seeking should continue to grow if favorable attitudes toward mental health professionals persist, mental health care remains accessible and affordable, and factors such as delayed age of marriage, high divorce rates, and job mobility lead many people to lead lives apart from strong social support groups. A vastly expanded mental health system ensures that voluntary help seeking is easier than ever before.

Despite the growth in help seeking from mental health professionals, a number of gaps remain between the needs of distressed people and the services available to them. One lies in the extent of help seeking for psychological problems in the general medical sector. Because many general medical providers are not sensitive to the needs of psychiatrically disordered persons, the treatment they dispense is often inadequate (Goldberg and Huxley, 1980). Mental health professionals must strive to work with primary-care providers so that psychiatric disorders will be recognized and treated appropriately within general medical practice.

Another major challenge for the mental health system in the 1990s will be to develop services that can meet the needs of chronic patients and their families without imposing undue involuntary control. Just as stringent commitment laws frustrate family efforts to seek help from inpatient

42

institutions, the organization of the mental health professions hinders the provision of outpatient treatment to chronic patients (Miller and Fiddleman, 1984; Peyrot, 1982). Mental health professionals obtain monetary, status, and reputational rewards for treating acute, well-off, and insightful patients (Schwartz, Krieger, and Sorenson, 1981). As a result, psychiatric caregivers resist working with chronic patients (Minkoff, 1987).

Services that would meet the needs of the seriously mentally ill and their families would be more encompassing and structured than traditional outpatient therapies but less restrictive than those found in custodial settings. There has been some progress in establishing halfway houses, sheltered care facilities, and day hospital treatments that meet the needs of specific chronic populations (Stein and Test, 1985). Some communities have established open facilities staffed by paraprofessionals who participate in and relate to the culture of young chronic patients. Others have established mobile units that bring services to persons on the street who would not otherwise seek them. Yet only a small number of such programs have developed that match appropriate treatment facilities with the needs of particular chronic populations.

Recent decades have seen dramatic alterations in both the sorts of conditions seen as amenable to psychiatric treatment and the nature of mental health systems. It will be particularly important to examine how help-seeking processes occur within a new organizational context. Changes in the nature of the mental health system and professions, as well as in patterns of help seeking, will be necessary if the provision of services is to match patient need.

References

Anderson, R., Francis, A., Lion, J., and Daughety, V. S. "Psychologically Related Illness and Health Services Utilization." *Medical Care,* 1977, *15,* 59–73.

Bachrach, L., Talbott, J. A., and Meyerson, A. T. "The Chronic Psychiatric Patient as a 'Difficult' Patient: A Conceptual Analysis." In A. T. Meyerson (ed.), *Barriers to Treating the Chronic Mentally Ill.* New Directions for Mental Health Services, no. 33. San Francisco: Jossey-Bass, 1987.

Balint, M. *The Doctor, His Patient, and the Illness.* New York: International Universities Press, 1957.

Clausen, J. A., Pfeffer, N. G., and Huffine, C. L. "Help Seeking in Severe Mental Illness." In D. Mechanic (ed.), *Symptoms, Illness Behavior, and Help Seeking.* New York: Neale Watson, 1982.

Clausen, J. A., and Yarrow, M. R. (eds.). "The Impact of Mental Illness on the Family." *The Journal of Social Issues,* 1955, *11* (entire issue).

Cleary, P. D. "New Directions in Illness Behavior Research." In S. McHugh and T. M. Vallis (eds.), *Illness Behavior: A Multidisciplinary Model.* New York: Plenum, 1986.

Fox, J. W. "Sex, Marital Status, and Age as Social Selection Factors in Recent Psychiatric Treatment." *Journal of Health and Social Behavior,* 1984, *25,* 394–405.

Freidson, E. *Profession of Medicine.* New York: Harper & Row, 1970.

Garrison, V. "Doctor, Espiritista, or Psychiatrist? Health-Seeking Behavior in a Puerto Rican Neighborhood of New York City." *Medical Anthropology*, 1977, *1* (entire issue).

George, L. K., Blazer, D. G., Winfield-Laird, I., Leaf, P. J., and Fischbach, R. L. "Psychiatric Disorders and Mental Health Service Use in Later Life: Evidence from the Epidemiological Catchment Area Program." Unpublished paper, 1987.

Gillis, L. S., and Keet, M. "Factors Underlying the Retention in the Community of Chronic Unhospitalized Schizophrenics." *British Journal of Psychiatry*, 1965, *111*, 1057-1067.

Ginsberg, S., and Brown, G. W. "No Time for Depression: A Study of Help Seeking Among Mothers of Preschool Children." In D. Mechanic (ed.), *Symptoms, Illness Behavior, and Help Seeking*. New York: Neale Watson, 1982.

Goldberg, D., and Huxley, P. *Mental Illness in the Community: The Pathway to Psychiatric Care*. London: Tavistock, 1980.

Gove, W. R., Tovo, M., and Hughes, M. "Involuntary Psychiatric Hospitalization: A Review of the Statutes Regulating the Social Control of the Mentally Ill." *Deviant Behavior*, 1985, *6*, 287-318.

Greenley, J. R., and Mechanic, D. "Social Selection in Seeking Help for Psychological Problems." *Journal of Health and Social Behavior*, 1976, *17*, 249-262.

Gurin, G., Veroff, J., and Field, S. *Americans View Their Mental Health*. New York: Basic Books, 1960.

Hollingshead, A. B., and Redlich, F. C. *Social Class and Mental Illness*. New York: Wiley, 1958.

Horwitz, A. "The Pathways into Psychiatric Treatment: Some Differences Between Men and Women." *Journal of Health and Social Behavior*, 1977a, *18*, 169-178.

Horwitz, A. "Social Networks and Pathways into Psychiatric Treatment." *Social Forces*, 1977b, *56*, 86-106.

Kadushin, C. *Why People Go to Psychiatrists*. New York: Atherton, 1969.

Kessler, R. C., Brown, R. L., and Broman, C. L. "Sex Differences in Psychiatric Help Seeking: Evidence from Four Large-Scale Surveys." *Journal of Health and Social Behavior*, 1981, *22*, 49-64.

Kramer, M. *Psychiatric Services and the Changing Institutional Scene, 1950-1985*. In National Institute of Mental Health, *Analytical and Special Study Reports*. Series B, no. 12. Washington, D.C.: U.S. Government Printing Office, 1977.

Leaf, P. J., and Bruce, M. L. "Gender Differences in the Use of Mental-Health-Related Services: A Reexamination." *Journal of Health and Social Behavior*, 1987, *28*, 171-183.

Leaf, P. J., Bruce, M. L., Tischler, G. L., Freeman, D. H., Weissman, M. M., and Myers, J. K. "Factors Affecting the Utilization of Specialty and General Medical Mental Health Services." Unpublished paper, 1987.

Leaf, P. J., Livingston, M. M., Tischler, G. L., Weissman, M. M., Holzer, C. E., and Myers, J. K. "Contact with Health Professionals for the Treatment of Psychiatric and Emotional Problems." *Medical Care*, 1985, *23*, 1322-1337.

Lerman, P. *Deinstitutionalization and the Welfare State*. New Brunswick, N.J.: Rutgers University Press, 1982.

Lin, T., Tardiff, K., Donetz, G., and Goresky, W. "Ethnicity and Patterns of Help Seeking." *Culture, Medicine, and Psychiatry*, 1978, *2*, 3-14.

Link, B., and Dohrenwend, B. P. "Formulation of Hypotheses about the Ratio of Untreated to Treated Cases in the True Prevalence Studies of Functional Psychiatric Disorders in Adults in the United States." In B. P. Dohrenwend, B. S.

44

Dohrenwend, M. S. Gould, B. Link, R. Neugebauer, and R. Wunsch-Hitzig (eds.), *Mental Illness in the United States: Epidemiological Estimates.* New York: Praeger, 1980.

Lowenthal, M. F. *Lives in Distress: The Paths of the Elderly to the Psychiatric War.* New York: Basic Books, 1964.

Marmor, J. *Psychiatrists and Their Patients: A National Study of Private Office Practice.* Washington, D.C.: American Psychiatric Association, 1975.

Mechanic, D. *Mental Health and Social Policy.* (2nd ed.). Englewood Cliffs, N.J.: Prentice-Hall, 1980.

Miller, R. D., and Fiddleman, P. B. "Outpatient Commitment: Treatment in the Least Restrictive Environment?" *Hospital and Community Psychiatry,* 1984, *35,* 147–151.

Minkoff, K. "Resistance of Mental Health Professionals to Working with the Chronic Mentally Ill." In A. T. Meyerson (ed.), *Barriers to Treating the Chronic Mentally Ill.* New Directions for Mental Health Services, no. 33. San Francisco: Jossey-Bass, 1987.

Morrissey, J. P., Tessler, R. C., and Farrin, L. L. "Being Seen But Not Admitted: A Note on Some Neglected Aspects of State Hospital Deinstitutionalization." *American Journal of Orthopsychiatry,* 1979, *49,* 153–156.

Myers, J. K., and Roberts, B. H. *Family and Class Dynamics in Mental Illness.* New York: Wiley, 1959.

National Institute of Mental Health. Unpublished data, 1987.

Pepper, B., and Ryglewicz, H. (eds.). *The Young Adult Chronic Patient.* New Directions for Mental Health Services, no. 14. San Francisco: Jossey-Bass, 1982.

Peyrot, M. "Caseload Management: Choosing Suitable Clients in a Community Health Clinic Agency." *Social Problems,* 1982, *30,* 157–167.

Robins, L. N., Helzer, J. E., Weissman, M. M., Orvaschel, H., Gruenberg, E., Burke, J. D., and Regier, D. A. "Lifetime Prevalence of Specific Psychiatric Disorders in Three Sites." *Archives of General Psychiatry,* 1984, *41,* 949–958.

Scheff, T. J. "Social Conditions for Rationality: How Urban and Rural Courts Deal with the Mentally Ill." *American Behavioral Scientist,* 1964, *7,* 21–24.

Schwartz, S. R., and Goldfinger, S. M. "The New Chronic Patient: Clinical Characteristics of an Emerging Subgroup." *Hospital and Community Psychiatry,* 1981, *32,* 470–474.

Schwartz, S., Krieger, M., and Sorenson, J. "Preliminary Survey of Therapists Who Work with Chronic Patients: Implications for Training." *Hospital and Community Psychiatry,* 1981, *32,* 799–800.

Segal, S. P., Baumohl, J., and Johnson, E. "Falling Through the Cracks: Mental Disorder and Social Margin in a Young Vagrant Population." *Social Problems,* 1977, *24,* 387–400.

Shapiro, S., Skinner, E. A., Kessler, L. G., Von Korff, M., German, P. S., Tischler, G. L., Leaf, P. J., Benham, L., Cottler, L., and Regier, D. A. "Utilization of Health and Mental Health Services." *Archives of General Psychiatry,* 1984, *41,* 971–978.

Srole, L., Langner, T. S., Michael, S. T., Opler, M. K., and Rennie, T.A.C. *Mental Health in the Metropolis: The Midtown Manhattan Study.* New York: McGraw-Hill, 1962.

Stein, L. I., and Test, M. A. (eds.). *The Training in Community Living Model: A Decade of Experience.* New Directions for Mental Health Services, no. 26. San Francisco: Jossey-Bass, 1985.

Stern, M. S. "Social Class and Psychiatric Treatment of Adults in the Mental Health Center." *Journal of Health and Social Behavior,* 1977, *18,* 317–325.

Taube, C. A., and Barrett, S. A. (eds.). *Mental Health, United States, 1985.* Washington, D.C.: U.S. Government Printing Office, 1985.

Tessler, R., Killian, L. M., and Gubman, G. D. "Stages in Family Response to Mental Illness: An Ideal Type." *Psychosocial Rehabilitation Journal,* 1987, *10,* 3-16.

Tessler, R., Mechanic, D., and Dimond, M. "The Effect of Psychological Distress on Physician Utilization: A Prospective Study." *Journal of Health and Social Behavior,* 1976, *19,* 253-264.

Tischler, G. L., Henisz, J. E., Myers, J. K., and Boswell, P. C. "Utilization of Mental Health Services." *Archives of General Psychiatry,* 1975, *32,* 411-415.

Tudor, W., Tudor, J. F., and Gove, W. R. "The Effect of Sex Role Differences on the Social Control of Mental Illness." *Journal of Health and Social Behavior,* 1977, *18,* 98-112.

Veroff, J., Kulka, R. A., and Douvan, E. *Mental Health in America: Patterns of Help Seeking from 1957 to 1976.* New York: Basic Books, 1981.

Allan V. Horwitz is associate professor and chairman of the Department of Sociology, Rutgers University. He is a member of the Institute for Health Care Policy, and Aging Research.

*Deinstitutionalization cannot improve the quality of life
of chronic mental patients unless mental health services
meet important needs, from basic subsistence to psychiatric
treatment and a regimen of activities. When properly
organized, services can also encourage social support, a
sense of mastery, self-esteem, coping skills, and incentives for
treatment.*

Services Organization and Quality of Life Among the Seriously Mentally Ill

Sarah Rosenfield

Deinstitutionalization of mental patients was accompanied by critiques of the destructive effects of institutional life. Criticisms focused on the social regression and the affronts to patients' sense of self in traditional mental hospitals (Goffman, 1961). Also, in adapting to institutional life, patients' ability to maneuver in the outside world eroded. Some critics have even argued that the debilitating effects of long-term custodial care were more damaging to mental health and well-being than the problems that required hospitalization in the first place (Rutman, 1976).

Improvement of patients' clinical condition and quality of life by the treatment and integration of patients within their own communities are major goals of the deinstitutionalization movement (Lamb, 1981; Bachrach, 1975; Beiser, Shore, Peters, and Tatum, 1985; Levine, 1987; Stein and Test, 1978; Lehman, Ward, and Linn, 1982; Lehman, 1983; Lehman, Possidente, and Hawker, 1986). Quality of life includes objective aspects such as the quality of the living situation, participation in social relations, leisure activities, and employment, as well as subjective aspects such as satisfaction with varying life dimensions. Wing (1978) states that "the quality of life lived by the patient is the final criterion by which services must be judged" (p. 254).

D. Mechanic (ed.). *Improving Mental Health Services: What the Social Sciences Can Tell Us.*
New Directions for Mental Health Services, no. 36. San Francisco: Jossey-Bass, 1987.

Critiques of Deinstitutionalization

For many patients, community-based treatment has neither improved their clinical condition nor their quality of life. Hospital stays are now shorter, but patients are often not connected to aftercare services following discharge and may receive little or no treatment in the community. Those who initially receive aftercare often drop out and are not reconnected to services (Rosenfield, 1986). The typically fragmented nature of community services adds to the problems for chronic patients, requiring that they negotiate among different agencies to receive needed services (Bachrach, 1975). Also, many community treatment programs have little interest in treating chronic patients whose prospects for improvement are limited and who are seen as generally unappealing. Such rejection is based in part on an acute care model of treatment that places little value on the goals of rehabilitation and maintenance characterizing the needs of the chronically mentally ill (Mechanic, 1986). Thus, while inpatient populations have declined in mental institutions over time, admission rates, particularly readmissions, have risen (Bassuk and Gerson, 1978). Specifically, between 35 and 50 percent of chronic mental patients are readmitted within one year of hospital discharge (Lamb, 1981; Anthony, Cohen, and Vitalo, 1978). As a result, there are questions about the accessibility and efficacy of community-based treatment.

Deinstitutionalization is criticized also for failing to improve the chronic patients' quality of life. Such patients often lack in basic needs such as food, clothing, housing, and medical care. Patients often live in substandard housing or, as low-cost housing is reduced in many areas, have become a substantial minority of the homeless population. Older patients and some young chronics are commonly in nursing homes, which offer custodial care without mental health treatment or appropriate staff (Mechanic, 1986). Also, chronic patients are typically unemployed and have trouble gaining competitive employment (Stein and Test, 1976). They are often socially isolated, with few social contacts and little participation in leisure activities (Lamb, 1981; Stein and Test, 1976; Mechanic, 1986). Community programs typically do not monitor these different needs, nor are they typically organized to address them. For these reasons, the ability of community-based treatment to improve patients' objective conditions and functioning as well as life satisfaction has been challenged.

Functions of Mental Hospitals

One explanation for the deficits of deinstitutionalization is the failure of community programs to reproduce some of the positive functions of the mental hospital in the community (Mechanic, 1986; Bachrach, 1975). Although effective treatment within total institutions was often problematic, hospitals provided crucial services to patients, which included psychiatric treatment, rehabilitation services, a regimen of activities, interpersonal contacts, and provisions for basic needs such as food, clothing, shelter, and medical care. Thus, if community care is to be humane and effective, it must provide these positive functions of the mental hospital.

There are several model programs of community-based treatment that have been successful in reducing rehospitalizations and improving the quality of life of chronic patients. Isolating the common elements that account for the success of these model systems points out some of the failures in community care more generally. In examining these elements, I also address the lack of sophisticated theories of intervention in the treatment of chronic patients (Mechanic, 1978). These model programs can serve as a basis for developing a systematic perspective to guide research and the organization of mental health services.

Model Community Programs

The Training in Community Living program in Madison, Wisconsin, is a widely known and effective model of community-based treatment (Stein and Test, 1976, 1978, 1980; Stein, Test, and Marx, 1975). Compared with controls randomly assigned to high-quality inpatient care, the patients in the community treatment group were rehospitalized less often and for less time and had fewer psychiatric symptoms. In terms of objective quality of life indicators, community treatment patients earned more from employment than controls, although they were no more often competitively employed. Community patients more frequently lived independently, although the quality of their living environments was no better. They had more contact with trusted friends and participated in social groups more often. In terms of subjective quality of life, patients in the community program were more satisfied with their lives, involving areas such as their living situation, friends, and work.

The Training in Community Living program diverts patients coming into the state hospital system, treats them, and teaches them coping skills within the community. Staff focus on teaching daily living skills (such as cooking and the use of public transportation), helping patients to find employment or sheltered workshop placement, and assisting them in learning social skills and using leisure time. Staff members accompany or stay with patients whenever needed. The program has two shifts of staff a day, with a staff member, in addition, on twenty-four-hour call. Aggressive outreach is done if patients do not show for work or other appointments. Medical status of patients is closely monitored.

This program was replicated in Sydney, Australia (New South Wales Department of Health, 1983). Patients from the state hospital were randomly assigned to the community project team or to standard inpatient care with community mental health center aftercare. The project team offered patients twenty-four-hour crisis services, intensive initial care, and individual counseling. The focus was also on training in basic living skills and social skills, family intervention, outreach when necessary, and monitoring of medical and other basic needs. Outcomes were similar to the Training in Community Living program. Rehospitalizations and symptoms were less for project-team patients than for controls. In addition, project-team patients perceived themselves to have greater coping ability than did controls. In terms of quality of life, project-team patients were more satisfied with their treatment; however, they did not have greater life satisfaction in general than controls. This contrast in satisfaction with participants in the Wisconsin program was attributed to the lower staff-patient ratio in the Australian project.

In a study of two community systems of care, treatment in the cities of Portland and Vancouver were contrasted (Beiser, Shore, Peters, and Tatum, 1985). The Vancouver program included outreach, individual programs for rehabilitation, twenty-four-hour emergency services, and close links among community resources. The Portland system resembled the more typical community care described at the beginning of this chapter. Vancouver patients were rehospitalized less, had fewer psychiatric symptoms, and reported a greater sense of well-being. They were also more often employed and more often satisfied with life.

These studies are the most comprehensive available in both program elements and evaluation of outcomes. In reducing rehospitalizations and improving quality of life in general, the program elements were effective. In each, project staff focus on psychiatric treatment and on rehabilitation in terms of daily living and social skills. Staff design a structure of activities for patients, including both work and leisure activities. The high staff-patient contact provides ongoing interpersonal relations. And basic human needs of housing, food, clothing, and medical care are monitored and arranged for.

Community systems that take responsibility for these elements of care are effective in enhancing quality of life. Even more limited programs focusing on some of these aspects are successful. Such programs include, for example, Fountain House, which is basically a job rehabilitation program (Beard, 1978; Beard, Malamud, and Rossman, 1978). Patients work in six areas of the clubhouse, such as the kitchen or clerical office, or in transitional employment in the community. Fountain House emphasizes the establishment of a familylike atmosphere. Staff follow up on members when they fail to attend. In addition, other services include leasing apartments for members. Fountain House members have lower rehospitalization rates and shorter lengths of stay than nonmembers, particularly when dropouts are followed up. The greater attendance fostered by the outreach program accounts for the lower rehospitalization rates.

The Soteria program is an alternative model of care for seriously mentally ill patients that takes an existential approach to psychosis with little use of medication (Mosher and Menn, 1978a, 1978b; Mosher and Keith, 1979). Soteria is a home for six residents and two nonprofessional staff with a surrogate-family atmosphere. Staff work intensively with patients within a nonhierarchical structure to give patients decision-making power. Comparing a small number of Soteria patients to similar patients in a community mental health center, rehospitalizations and symptoms are somewhat less among Soteria patients. In relation to objective quality of life, Soteria patients are more often living independently than control patients. They are also significantly better in psychosocial adjustment (for example, in interpersonal relations) than controls. Although there are no differences in the numbers working, Soteria patients showed increases in occupational status over a two-year period more often than did the controls.

In Philadelphia, nonprofessional community members called enablers are used in a home treatment program (Weinman and Kleiner, 1978). Enablers stay in contact with patients along with professional counselors who teach daily living skills. Some patients also live with enablers. Patients treated by enablers have been compared to those receiving standard inpatient treatment as well as to inpatients receiving a form of socioenvironmental therapy similar to the experimental group. Those in the enabler program were somewhat lower in rehospitalizations at one year follow-up, although no different in symptoms. Self-esteem improved for experimental patients more than for controls over time. Social contacts and instrumental performance (such as shopping and cooking) improved for enabler patients more than for inpatients receiving socio-environmental therapy but were not different from traditional ward patients. The lack of improvement over ward patients was attributed to the dropout rates of the more seriously ill patients in the ward setting, leaving only higher functioning patients for comparison with the experimental group.

In the lodge society program, patients move in small groups into the community (Fairweather, 1978). They establish their own governing body for decision making and use staff solely as consultants. In one case, patients developed their own business and became successfully self-supporting. Compared to a standard inpatient care group over four years, lodge society patients were less often rehospitalized. They were also more often employed, more satisfied with work, and reported greater personal enhancement.

Intervening Factors

In sum, successful community programs have in common the provision of basic needs, treatment and rehabilitation, a regimen of activities, and interpersonal contacts. Such functions obviously assist patients in very direct ways. However, I suggest that these functions, and thus these program elements, also provide five crucial factors that are positive for mental status and quality of life in general and for chronic patients in particular. These intervening factors include the provision of social support, self-esteem, mastery or control, coping ability, and incentives to treatment.

Social Support. Psychiatric treatment, rehabilitation, and interpersonal contacts provide a basis for social support. Although social support includes help with practical problems and sociability, emotional support is most often emphasized in relation to well-being. In addition, although social support has been conceptualized in terms of the number of social relationships (or social integration) and the structure of relationships (or social networks), the functional content or what people get from social relationships is considered to be the most precise meaning of support (House, 1987). Thus, we can define social support as "the subjective feeling of belonging, of being accepted, of being loved, of being needed all for oneself and not for what one can do" (Moss, 1973, p. 237).

The importance of social support in general populations has been widely documented. Social support improves mental health status both directly and by buffering the effects of stressful events (Thoits, 1982; Heller and Swindle, 1983; Kessler, Price, and Wortman, 1985; Shumaker and Brownell, 1984). Social support is particularly effective in combatting the salient problems of the seriously mentally ill. Schizophrenic patients, for example, have difficulty forming and maintaining relationships and thus serious problems with social isolation (Mechanic, 1978; Torrey, 1986; New South Wales Department of Health, 1983; Bachrach, 1981). Chronic patients continue to have these social deficits even when their symptoms are controlled by drugs (Liberman, Mueser, and Wallace, 1986). Evidence shows that social support affects rehospitalizations, social functioning, and the subjective evaluation of quality of life among the seriously mentally ill (Grusky and others, 1986; Lehman, 1983). Specifically, supportiveness of family members—as opposed to "expressed emotion" characterized by critical communications and intrusiveness—lowers the chance of relapse among schizophrenic patients (Brown, Monck, Carstairs, and Wing, 1962; Vaughn and Leff, 1976; Goldstein, 1983; Goldstein and Doane, 1982). Further, interventions with families that lower expressed emotion can reduce patient relapse rate (Boyd, McGill, and Falloon, 1981).

The provision of social support is evidenced in the treatment and rehabilitation functions in the model programs described. Moreover, the provision of this support is used to explain the successes in some programs and the failures in others. Mosher and Menn (1978a) claim that Soteria works without medication because the nurturant atmosphere operates as a substitute. Less social support (in terms of less staff-patient contact) in the Australian model of the Training in Community Living program resulted in more social isolation, less satisfaction with social relations, and thus less life satisfaction for the Australian patients (New South Wales Department of Health, 1983). Finally, the lack of social support as measured by conflict between patients and staff resulted in negative outcomes for chronic patients in the enabler program (Weinman and Kleiner, 1978).

Mosher and Keith (1979) note that much group work with seriously ill patients is directed toward providing social support. They state that "the most effective types of psychosocial treatment for schizophrenia are those that provide the most comprehensive, corrective, sustaining social support systems" (p. 629).

Mastery. Treatment and rehabilitation, particularly socialization programs, as well as interpersonal contacts, raise patients' sense of mastery or control. Several theoretical perspectives link perceptions of control—in terms of learned helplessness, locus of control, fatalism, or mastery—to symptoms. For example, research shows that beliefs in external control—that is, that events and rewards depend on forces outside the individual such as luck or fate versus one's own qualities or behavior— are related to symptomatology (Rotter, 1966; Mirowsky and Ross, 1984; Leggett and Archer, 1979; Abramowitz, 1969; Calhoun, Cheney, and Davies, 1974; Evans, 1981; Costello, 1982; Phares, 1962). Arguments on fatalism (Kohn, 1972) connect the perception that one is "at the mercy of forces and people beyond one's control" (p. 300) to schizophrenia, anxiety, and depression (Wheaton, 1980, 1983). Mastery is described as a basic goal of self-enhancement that helps protect the self against threats (Pearlin, Lieberman, Menaghan, and Mullan, 1981). Its loss is thus a "final step in the process leading to stress" (p. 340).

Perceptions of low mastery or lack of self-determination result directly in feelings of helplessness and hopelessness and thus affect individuals' sense of well-being. The inability to affect one's environment also results in feelings of personal failure (Rosenfield, 1987). Further, attributing causation to forces outside oneself gives individuals less flexibility in reacting to stressful situations and less motivation for coping efforts in general (Thoits, 1987). A fatalistic outlook leads to a fearful view of the world and thus limits options for action (Kohn, 1972). When the point of coping efforts is unclear, there is less reason for and thus less persistence in coping behavior (Wheaton, 1980, 1983).

Chronic patients are particularly vulnerable to perceptions of low mastery. Seriously mentally ill patients often have the sense of being overwhelmed and of being powerless victims of a disease over which they have little control. They feel in general at the mercy of all-powerful forces outside of themselves and thus lack a sense of control over their symptoms as well as the demands of their environment (Lamb, 1982; Mosher and Menn, 1978b; Mendel and Allen, 1978). Increased control is related to greater social activity, greater happiness, and lower mortality rates among nursing home populations (Rodin and Langer, 1977; Rodin, 1986), suggesting its relevance for chronic patients.

Patients gain a sense of competence and mastery in the model programs through learning daily living skills (some emphasizing employment and others both employment and other skills) or through the structure of the treatment setting itself, such as the nonhierarchical Soteria model and the self-governing lodge society. In sum, to give chronic patients a greater sense of mastery, mental health services should focus on a rehabilitation model of mental illness as opposed to a medical model, with the objective of returning a sense of self-determination to chronic patients (Mendel and Allen, 1978).

Self-Esteem. Partly by improving social support and mastery, the service elements of psychiatric treatment, rehabilitation, and interpersonal contacts raise patients' sense of self-esteem. Certainly, we know that the lack of a sense of mastery and inadequate social support erode self-esteem (Lamb, 1982; Mosher and Menn, 1978a; Mendel and Allen, 1978; Pearlin, Lieberman, Menaghan, and Mullan, 1981). Low levels of self-esteem are linked to high symptoms in response to life events in general (Pearlin and Schooler, 1978; Kessler, 1982). Further, low self-esteem, or self-derogation, results in high symptoms and poor social functioning among chronic patients in particular. High self-derogation predicts impaired functioning and high symptom and rehospitalization rates among chronic patients discharged from hospitals (Lorimor, Kaplan, and Pokorny, 1985). Thus, program elements that enhance self-esteem lower recidivism and improve functioning for seriously mentally ill patients.

Coping Ability. Chronic patients are particularly vulnerable to stress because they have a limited repertoire of coping skills. Such disabilities lead to problems with work habits, social relations, and leisure activities, which constitute patients' quality of life (Test, 1979; Stein, Test, and Marx, 1975). Further, the way individuals respond to stress, whether by changing the problem, changing the interpretation of the problem, or managing the distress caused by the problem, has significant consequences for mental health symptoms (Folkman and Lazarus, 1980; Pearlin and Schooler, 1978; Kessler, 1985). Different coping strategies are more effective for varying areas of strain (Pearlin and Schooler, 1978). Thus, programs that expand options and skills for coping reduce symptoms and improve quality of life for chronic patients.

Incentives for Treatment. Finally, the structure of activities as well as the support from treatment and rehabilitation programs encourage participation in treatment. A major problem among chronic patients is a lack of motivation not only for treatment but also for engagement in social life and leisure activities (Stein and Test, 1978). Patients who do not attend treatment programs or who attend less frequently are rehospitalized more often than those receiving consistent aftercare treatment (Pasamanick, Scarpetti, and Dinitz, 1967; Hogarty and Goldberg, 1973; Byers, Cohen, and Harshbarger, 1978; Serban, 1980; Sands, 1984). The social support provided in treatment and rehabilitation programs encourages patients to participate in treatment and social activities as well as to feel they are not alone (Stein and Test, 1978). By motivating patients to engage in treatment and in social life in general, such programs improve patients' mental status and quality of life.

Conclusion

The failure of deinstitutionalization to improve the quality of life of chronic mental patients is due to the absence in many community programs of the positive functions typically served by mental hospitals. Fulfilling basic human needs and providing treatment, rehabilitation, interpersonal contacts, and a regimen of activities are important beyond their obvious immediate value. Indirect effects include the enhancement of social support, self-esteem, mastery, coping skills, and incentives for treatment. Community-based systems appear to be effective insofar as they respond to patients' basic functional needs and trigger these intervening factors.

The explanatory model proposed here is multivariate; functions, intervening variables, and outcomes are linked both directly and indirectly. For example, rehabilitation is directly linked to employment, but it also enhances the patient's social support and mastery, which in turn improve quality of life and lower the rate of rehospitalization through their impact on self-esteem and coping ability.

Evaluators of model systems often note that they do not know which program elements are responsible for their successful outcomes (Stein and Test, 1978; New South Wales Department of Health, 1983). This analysis suggests the reasons for the effectiveness of these elements. However, future research needs to test this explanatory framework and identify clearly which intervening variables are most responsible for specific outcomes.

References

Abramowitz, S. "Locus of Control and Self-Reported Depression Among College Students." *Psychological Reports,* 1969, 25, 149-150.

Anthony, W. A., Cohen, M. R., and Vitalo, R. "The Measurement of Rehabilitative Outcome." *Schizophrenia Bulletin*, 1978, *4*, 365–383.

Bachrach, L. L. *Deinstitutionalization: An Analytical Review and Sociological Perspective*. Washington, D.C.: U.S. Department of Health, Education, and Welfare, 1975.

Bachrach, L. L. "Continuity of Care for Chronic Mental Patients: A Conceptual Analysis." *American Journal of Psychiatry*, 1981, *138*, 1449–1456.

Bassuk, E., and Gerson, S. "Deinstitutionalization and Mental Health Services." *Scientific American*, 1978, *238*, 46–56.

Beard, J. H. "The Rehabilitation Services of Fountain House." In L. I. Stein, and M. A. Test (eds.), *Alternatives to Mental Hospital Treatment*. New York: Plenum, 1978.

Beard, J. H., Malamud, T. J., and Rossman, E. "Psychiatric Rehabilitation and Long-Term Rehospitalization Rates: The Findings of Two Research Studies." *Schizophrenia Bulletin*, 1978, *4*, 622–635.

Beiser, M., Shore, J. H., Peters, R., and Tatum, E. "Does Community Care for the Mentally Ill Make a Difference? A Tale of Two Cities." *American Journal of Psychiatry*, 1985, *142*, 1047–1052.

Boyd, J. L., McGill, C. W., Falloon, I.R.H. "Family Participation in the Community Rehabilitation of Schizophrenics." *Hospital and Community Psychiatry*, 1981, *32*, 629–632.

Brown, G. W., Monck, E. M., Carstairs, G. M., and Wing, J. K. "The Influence of Family Life on the Course of Schizophrenia." *British Journal of Preventive Social Medicine*, 1962, *16*, 55–68.

Byers, E. S., Cohen, S., and Harshbarger, D. D. "Impact of Aftercare Services on Recidivism of Mental Hospital Patients." *Community Health Journal*, 1978, *14*, 26–34.

Calhoun, L., Cheney, T., and Davies, S. "Locus of Control, Self-Reported Depression, and Perceived Causes of Depression." *Journal of Consulting Psychology*, 1974, *42*, 736–745.

Costello, E. "Locus of Control and Depression in Students and Psychiatric Outpatients." *Journal of Clinical Psychology*, 1982, *36*, 661–667.

Evans, R. "The Relationship of Two Measures of Perceived Control to Depression." *Journal of Personality Assessment*, 1981, *45*, 66–70.

Fairweather, G. "The Development, Evaluation, and Diffusion of Rehabilitative Programs: A Social Change Process." In L. I. Stein, and M. A. Test (eds.), *Alternatives to Mental Hospital Treatment*. New York: Plenum, 1978.

Folkman, S., and Lazarus, R. S. "An Analysis of Coping in a Middle-Aged Community Sample." *Journal of Health and Social Behavior*, 1980, *21*, 219–239.

Goffman, E. *Asylums: Essays on the Social Situation of Mental Patients and Other Inmates*. New York: Doubleday, 1961.

Goldstein, M. J. "Family Interaction: Patterns Predictive of the Onset and Course of Schizophrenia." In H. Steirlin, L. C. Wynne, and M. Wirsching (eds.), *Psychosocial Interventions in Schizophrenia*. New York: Springer-Verlag, 1983.

Goldstein, M. J., and Doane, J. A. "Family Factors in the Onset, Course, and Treatment of Schizophrenia Spectrum Disorders: An Update on Current Research." *Journal of Nervous and Mental Disorder*, 1982, *170*, 692–700.

Grusky, O., Tierney, K., Manderscheid, R. W., and Grusky, D. B. "Social Bonding and Community Adjustment of Chronically Mentally Ill Adults." *Journal of Health and Social Behavior*, 1986, *26*, 49–63.

Heller, K., and Swindle, R. "Social Networks, Perceived Social Support, and Coping with Stress." In R. D. Felner, L. S. Jason, J. Moritsugu, and S. S. Farber (eds.), *Prevention Psychology: Theory, Research, and Practice in Community Intervention.* Elmsford, New York: Pergamon Press, 1983.

Hogarty, G. E., and Goldberg, S. L. "Collaborative Study Group: Drug and Sociotherapy in Aftercare of Schizophrenic Patients: One-Year Relapse Rates." *Archives of General Psychiatry,* 1973, *28,* 54-64.

House, J. "Social Support and Social Structure." *Sociological Forum,* 1987, *2,* 135-146.

Kessler, R. C. "A Disaggregation of the Relationship Between Socioeconomic Status and Psychological Distress." *American Sociological Review,* 1982, *47,* 752-764.

Kessler, R. C., Price, R. H., and Wortman, C. "Social Factors in Psychopathology: Stress, Social Support, and Coping Processes." *Annual Review of Psychology,* 1985, *36,* 531-572.

Kohn, M. "Class, Family, and Schizophrenia." *Social Forces,* 1972, *50,* 295-302.

Lamb, H. R. "What Did We Really Expect from Deinstitutionalization?" *Hospital and Community Psychiatry,* 1981, *32,* 105-109.

Lamb, H. R. *Treating the Long-Term Mentally Ill.* San Francisco: Jossey-Bass, 1982.

Leggett, J., and Archer, R. "Locus of Control and Depression Among Psychiatric Inpatients." *Psychological Reports,* 1979, *45,* 835-838.

Lehman, A. F. "The Well-Being of Chronic Mental Patients: Assessing Their Quality of Life." *Archives of General Psychiatry,* 1983, *40,* 369-373.

Lehman, A., Possidente, S., and Hawker, F. "The Quality of Life of Chronic Patients in a State Hospital and in Community Residences." *Hospital and Community Psychiatry,* 1986, *37,* 901-907.

Lehman, A. F., Ward, N., and Linn, L. "Chronic Mental Patients: The Quality of Life Issue." *American Journal of Psychiatry,* 1982, *139,* 1271-1276.

Levine, S. "The Changing Terrains in Medical Sociology: Emergent Concern with Quality of Life." *Journal of Health and Social Behavior,* 1987, *28,* 1-6.

Liberman, R. P., Mueser, K. T., and Wallace, C. J. "Social Skills Training for Schizophrenic Individuals at Risk for Relapse." *American Journal of Psychiatry,* 1986, *143,* 523-526.

Lorimor, R. J., Kaplan, H. B., and Pokorny, A. D. "Self-Derogation and Adjustment in the Community: A Longitudinal Study of Psychiatric Patients." *American Journal of Psychiatry,* 1985, *142,* 1442-1446.

Mechanic, D. "Alternatives to Mental Hospital Treatment: A Sociological Perspective." In L. I. Stein, and M. A. Test (eds.), *Alternatives to Mental Hospital Treatment.* New York: Plenum, 1978.

Mechanic, D. "The Challenge of Chronic Mental Illness: A Retrospective and Prospective View." *Hospital and Community Psychiatry,* 1986, *37,* 891-896.

Mendel, W. M., and Allen, R. E. "Rescue and Rehabilitation." In L. I. Stein, and M. A. Test (eds.), *Alternatives to Mental Hospital Treatment.* New York: Plenum, 1978.

Mirowsky, J., and Ross, C. E. "Mexican Culture and Its Emotional Contradictions." *Journal of Health and Social Behavior,* 1984, *25,* 2-13.

Mosher, L. R., and Keith, S. J. "Research on the Psychosocial Treatment of Schizophrenia: A Summary Report." *American Journal of Psychiatry,* 1979, *136,* 623-631.

Mosher, L. R., and Menn, A. Z. "Community Residential Treatment for Schizophrenia: Two-Year Follow-Up." *Hospital and Community Psychiatry,* 1978a, *29,* 715-723.

Mosher, L. R., and Menn, A. Z. "Lowered Barriers in the Community: The Soteria Model." In L. I. Stein, and M. A. Test (eds.), *Alternatives to Mental Hospiital Treatment*. New York: Plenum, 1978b.

Moss, G. *Illness, Immunity, and Social Interaction*. New York: Wiley, 1973.

New South Wales Department of Health. *Psychiatric Hospital versus Community Treatment: A Controlled Study*. Sydney, Australia: New South Wales, Department of Health, 1983.

Pasamanick, B., Scarpetti, F. R., and Dinitz, S. *Schizophrenia in the Community*. New York: Appleton-Century-Crofts, 1967.

Pearlin, L. I., Lieberman, M. A., Menaghan, E. G., and Mullan, J. T. "The Stress Process." *Journal of Health and Social Behavior*, 1981, *22*, 337–356.

Pearlin, L., and Schooler, C. "The Structure of Coping." *Journal of Health and Social Behavior*, 1978, *19*, 2–21.

Phares, E. J. "Perceptual Threshold Decrements as a Function of Skill and Chance Experiences." *Journal of Psychology*, 1962, *53*, 399–407.

Rodin, J. "Aging and Health: Effects of the Sense of Control." *Science*, 1986, *233*, 1271–1276.

Rodin, J., and Langer, E. "Long-Term Effects of a Control-Relevant Intervention with the Institutionalized Aged." *Journal of Personality and Social Psychology*, 1977, *35*, 897–902.

Rosenfield, S. "Closing the Gaps: Evaluation of a Linking Program from the Hospital to the Community for Chronic Mental Patients." *Journal of Applied Behavioral Science*, 1986, *22*, 411–423.

Rosenfield, S. "The Effects of Women's Employment: Personal Control and Sex Differences in Mental Health." Unpublished manuscript, 1987.

Rotter, J. B. "Generalized Expectancies for Internal Versus External Control of Reinforcement." *Psychological Monographs*, 1966, *80*, 1–28.

Rutman, I. D. *Adequate Residential Community-Based Program for the Mentally Disabled*. Philadelphia: Horizon House Institute, 1976.

Sands, R. G. "Correlates of Success and Lack of Success in Deinstitutionalization." *Community Mental Health Journal*, 1984, *20*, 223–235.

Serban, G. *Adjustment of Schizophrenics in the Community*. New York: S. P. Medical and Scientific Books, 1980.

Shumaker, S. A., and Brownell, A. "Toward a Theory of Social Support: Closing Conceptual Gaps." *Journal of Social Issues*, 1984, *40*, 11–36.

Stein, L. L., and Test, M. A. "Training in Community Living: A Follow-Up Look at a Gold-Award Program." *Hospital and Community Psychiatry*, 1976, *27*, 193–194.

Stein, L. I., and Test, M. A. "Training in Community Living: Research Design and Results." In L. I. Stein, and M. A. Test (eds.), *Alternatives to Mental Hospital Treatment*. New York: Plenum, 1978.

Stein, L. I., and Test, M. A. "Alternative to Mental Hospital Treatment." *Archives of General Psychiatry*, 1980, *37*, 392–397.

Stein, L. I., Test, M. A., and Marx, A. J. "Alternative to the Hospital: A Controlled Study." *American Journal of Psychiatry*, 1975, *132*, 517–522.

Test, M. A. "Continuity of Care in Community Treatment." In L. I. Stein (ed.), *Community Support Systems for the Long-Term Patient*. New Directions for Mental Health Services, no. 2. San Francisco: Jossey-Bass, 1979.

Thoits, P. A. "Conceptual, Methodological, and Theoretical Problems in Studying Social Support as a Buffer Against Life Stress." *Journal of Health and Social Behavior*, 1982, *23*, 145–159.

Thoits, P. A. "Gender and Marital Status Differences in Control and Distress:

Common Stress Versus Unique Stress Explanations." *Journal of Health and Social Behavior*, 1987, *28*, 7-22.

Torrey, E. F. "Continuous Treatment Teams in the Care of the Chronically Mentally Ill." *Hospital and Community Psychiatry*, 1986, *37*, 1243-1247.

Vaughn, C. E., and Leff, J. P. "The Influence of Family and Social Factors on the Course of Psychiatric Illness: A Comparison of Schizophrenic and Depressed Neurotic Patients." *British Journal of Psychiatry*, 1976, *129*, 125-137.

Weinman, B., and Kleiner, R. J. "The Impact of Community Living and Community Member Intervention on the Adjustment of the Chronically Psychotic Patient." In L. I. Stein, and M. A. Test (eds.), *Alternatives to Mental Hospital Treatment*. New York: Plenum, 1978.

Wheaton, B. "The Sociogenesis of Psychological Disorder: An Attributional Theory." *Journal of Health and Social Behavior*, 1980, *21*, 100-124.

Wheaton, B. "Stress, Personal Coping Resources, and Psychiatric Symptoms: An Investigation of Interactive Models." *Journal of Health and Social Behavior*, 1983, *24*, 208-229.

Wing, J. W. "Planning and Evaluating Services for Chronically Handicapped Psychiatric Patients in the United Kingdom." In L. I. Stein, and M. A. Test (eds.), *Alternatives to Mental Hospital Treatment*. New York: Plenum, 1978.

Sarah Rosenfield is assistant professor of sociology and member of the Institute of Health, Health Care Policy, and Aging Research, Rutgers University.

*Case managers must balance the interests of the service
delivery system with the demands of their relationships with
clients. This dual allegiance has problematic consequences for
the design and practice of case management for the chronically
mentally ill.*

Issues in Case Management for
the Chronically Mentally Ill

Ann E. P. Dill

Although its antecedents date to social service exchanges organized in the
nineteenth century, case management for the chronically mentally ill has
become a fixture in the mental health system only within the past decade.
The impetus came largely from the National Standards for Community
Mental Health Centers and the inauguration of the National Institute of
Mental Health (NIMH) Community Support Program (CSP) (Levine
and Fleming, 1986; Platman and others, 1982).

Studies of CSP demonstration sites have addressed numerous issues
concerning the design and practice of case management (Intagliata and
Baker, 1983; Stroul, 1984). The current expansion of similar programs to
new mental health settings increases the need for consensus and clarity
about the nature of the case manager role and the functions it serves
(Goldstrom and Manderscheid, 1983; Harrod, 1986). This chapter uses
sociological theory to elucidate the dilemmas inherent in the case manager role due to its function as an intermediary between formal organizations and clients.

Theoretical Perspective

The organization of social life takes place through two essential
but opposite structures: primary groups, such as kin, friends, and neigh-

D. Mechanic (ed.). *Improving Mental Health Services: What the Social Sciences Can Tell Us.*
New Directions for Mental Health Services, no. 36. San Francisco: Jossey-Bass, 1987.

bors, and formal organizations, of which the archetype is the bureaucracy. As characterized by Weber (1947), attributes of the bureaucracy include: a high level of specialization and division of labor; coordination through rules and hierarchy; appointment and evaluation based on technical criteria and merit; impersonal motivation of members through economic incentives; and social relations in large groups based primarily on instrumental ties and time-limited commitment.

The features of primary groups represent the antithesis to each of those attributes (Cooley, 1909). Thus, ties among primary-group members are diffuse, relating to diverse aspects of daily life. Personal contact is required for primary groups to function; recruitment and evaluation are individualistic and affective. Social relations take place in small groups with long-term, even permanent, commitment, and identification with the group is the main source of a member's motivation.

Although primary groups and formal organizations have opposing structures, current social research shows that they may complement, rather than oppose, one another and may, indeed, be most effective in the presence of each other. One theoretical framework posits that primary groups and formal organizations can both be optimally effective when each manages tasks that best match its structural characteristics (Litwak, 1985): in other words, formal organizations are most effective when technical knowledge is involved and when tasks can be routinized or simplified through a division of labor. In contrast, because of the face-to-face contact, diffuse affective relations, and long-term commitment of primary groups, they are more effective at handling unpredictable and contingency-laden events, as well as tasks that cannot be subdivided.

The analysis that follows will examine the consequences of combining attributes characteristic of primary groups with those of formal organizations within the same social role—namely, that of case manager.

Case Management as Formal Organization and as Primary Group

Case managers function as "the human link between the client and the system" (Intagliata, 1982, p. 659). As this image suggests, case managers maintain relations that resemble those of a primary group with clients, while at the same time functioning as members of formal organizations within the service system. The objectives of case management are, in fact, responses to difficulties within that system: "Case management is essentially a problem-solving function designed to ensure continuity of services and to overcome system rigidity, fragmented services, and misutilization of certain facilities, and inaccessibility" (Joint Commission on the Accreditation of Hospitals, 1976, p. 21).

Although they are usually set in agencies with a "human relations" rather than a "bureaucratic" orientation (Litwak, 1985), case management programs have many of the characteristics of bureaucracies. These include a status hierarchy, governance by formal rules and standards, impersonal recruitment and evaluation, and an economically based reward system. Case management in these programs plays a specialized role; in addition, the functions of case management may themselves form a basis for specialization, as when each member of a team of case managers assumes particular expertise in, for example, entitlements or client residential placement (Levine and Fleming, 1986).

Because they occupy a position that connects organizations, as well as organizations and clients, case managers serve as organizational "boundary spanners" (Aldrich and Herker, 1977). To be able to integrate various services, case managers must be invested with some degree of organizational authority, whether formal, such as interagency agreements, or informal, such as working relationships backed by mutual collegial respect (Schwartz, Goldman, and Churgin, 1982; Kanter, 1985).

While the connection of case management to formal organizations is thus quite clear, characterizing it as having features of primary groups may seem metaphorical. Indeed, the case manager's relation to clients is often compared to that of "friend," "parent," "older brother or sister," or even "ego"—the ultimate primary-group member (Baker and Weiss, 1984; Harris and Bergman, 1987; Kanter, 1985; Levine, 1979).

What these metaphors convey is the diffuse responsibility attached to case management, the extensive one-to-one contact between case manager and client, the focus on problems in everyday living, and the long-term commitment case management programs make to clients. The last reflects, as well, the organizational context of case management (that is, the organization and its tasks endure even if individual staff members leave); nonetheless, it and the other properties mentioned are precisely those that are characteristic of primary groups.

Two sets of issues will now be considered that reveal consequences of this combination of organizational and primary-group properties in case management.

Role Conflict in Case Management

Although it is possible to speak of the "case manager role," case managers may perform an array of roles to differing degrees, depending on the nature of service systems and client needs. Among these are: diagnostician, counselor, planner, service expediter and provider, record keeper, client advocate, caseload manager, and community organizer (Kemp, 1981).

These roles compete for the case manager's time and priority; moreover, the requirements and responsibilities of some roles can conflict with those of others. For example, representing clients to other service agencies may require the case manager to assume the assertiveness of a salesperson—a stance that may be inappropriate in counseling relation-ships with clients (Kemp, 1981). The multiple and conflicting demands of case managers' roles often lead to staff burnout and turnover (Intagli-ata and Baker, 1983; Minnesota Community Support Project, 1980).

Underlying the role conflicts faced by case managers are differing expectations regarding their activities held by their own organizations, by other service agencies, and by clients and their families (Harrod, 1986; Mueller and Hopp, 1987). While conflicts of interest may occur between (or even within) any of these "constituencies," several issues arise specif-ically because case management is governed both by the standards of formal organizations and by the need to maintain primary-group-like ties to clients.

One such issue concerns the confidentiality accorded client infor-mation. The many and diffuse relations between case managers and clients yield equally diverse types of information. This information is important for the case manager in establishing a complete and integrated perspective on the client's life (Levine and Fleming, 1986). Sharing that information and perspective with other agencies can enhance the case manager's ability to integrate the service system on behalf of the client (Test, 1979); it may also, however, threaten the client's privacy or be perceived by the client as a violation of interpersonal trust. Ensuring confidentiality to clients can be accomplished through several organiza-tional and legal mechanisms (Wolowitz, 1983); in daily practice, however, situations will still arise in which the case manager must make a more subtle adjudication, balancing the needs of service agencies with the sanctity of the relationship to the client (Diamond and Wikler, 1985). What, for example, should be a case manager's response to learning that a client has misrepresented himself or herself to another agency because, in the client's experience, telling "the truth" leads to a denial of services (Kanter, 1985; Levine, 1979)?

Client advocacy is a second function particularly affected by the combination of organizational and primary-group attributes in case man-agement. Like the client's family and friends, case managers are allied to the client's cause in receiving needed services; however, since most ser-vices are funded or provided by the state, case managers who are public employees face "an obvious conflict of interest when they have to advo-cate on behalf of a client against their employer" (Wolowitz, 1983, p. 83). Proposed solutions to this situation have included removing case man-agement from the state mental health system (Platman and others, 1982) or making the advocacy role independent of case management programs (Wolowitz, 1983).

A final problematic aspect of the case manager's role concerns the case manager's use of authority. Clients' perceptions of case managers' trustworthiness and personal dedication may be undermined when case managers act as agents of the mental health system—for example, by instituting involuntary commitment proceedings. Organizational authority is invested in case managers in more subtle ways as well, such as their ability to decide what information to give to clients about the service system (Kanter, 1985).

Such inherent power differentials may be at odds with case management objectives of working with clients on a more collaborative basis, respecting their preferences, and promoting their autonomy (Kanter, 1985; Wolowitz, 1983). These issues may be especially critical in the care of younger chronic patients, who constitute the fastest-growing segment of the clientele of case management programs (Berzon and Lowenstein, 1984).

The different and conflicting demands that arise because case managers must respond to organizational interests as well as those of their clients can cause problems in the course of the case manager's everyday practice. For example, some case managers may emphasize one aspect of their role at the expense of the other. Kurtz, Bagarozzi, and Pollane (1984) found that case managers in community mental health centers seldom performed activities that required working with staff at other agencies; instead, they emphasized those that kept them in contact with clients.

Similarly, Caragonne (1980) found that, when case managers lacked clarity about their roles, they were more likely to give clients direct services involving personal contact, such as counseling, than to spend time on such activities as service linkage and monitoring. Interestingly, the case managers' supervisors and administrators assumed that their staff were spending more time on the latter activities and underestimated the amount of time they spent on direct services. These studies suggest that case managers may be drawn more to the primary-group aspects of their work than to formal organizational functions and that supervisory structures must ensure that such preferential orientations do not lead to the neglect of service linkages essential to maintaining clients in the community.

It is also likely that case managers have developed their own strategies for balancing the organizational demands of their roles with their relations to clients, rather than trading one off against the other. Baker and Weiss (1984), for example, found that CSP case managers avoided role conflict by negotiating between clients and treatment teams, interpreting for each the actions and beliefs of the other. Further research is needed to elucidate such adaptive strategies and to evaluate their relative effectiveness in enhancing case managers' performance and client outcomes.

Attributes of Case Managers and Their Programs

A second set of issues related to the combination of bureaucratic and primary-group properties concerns the structure of case management programs and the qualifications of case managers.

Many of the functions of case management involve relatively standardized tasks that require specialized knowledge of the service system; examples are entitlement assessment and interagency referral. The more general objective of integrating services for clients requires, as well, a focus on the systems level. It is generally recognized, however, that "case management alone simply cannot be expected to solve the problems created by incomplete, inadequate service systems" (Intagliata and Baker, 1983, p. 87). Furthermore, the very problems in the system that create the need for case management programs, such as lack of interagency coordination, can impede the effectiveness of those programs (Caragonne, 1980; Kurtz, Bagarozzi, and Pollane, 1984).

The standardized nature of some case management tasks, the system-level focus of case management objectives, and the recurrent problems characteristic of mental health service systems suggest that formal integration mechanisms need to be placed at a higher administrative level than that provided by case management (Litwak, 1985). For example, the demonstration projects sponsored by the Robert Wood Foundation and the U.S. Department of Housing and Urban Development have established municipal authorities to centralize administrative and fiscal responsibility for social as well as mental health services (Mechanic, 1986). The need remains, however, for integration of services at the client level: Today's clients can't wait for tomorrow's program.

Strategies for improving the ability of case management programs to mobilize the service system for clients generally involve modifications in the organizational structure of those programs, such as increased task specialization or the introduction of standardized coordination mechanisms. The use of paraprofessional case management aides for clerical linkage and monitoring routines illustrates task specialization (Levine and Fleming, 1986); interagency service agreements exemplify formal coordination mechanisms (Altman, 1982; Intagliata and Baker, 1983), of which the epitome may be computerized client-tracking systems and management algorithms (Friday, 1986; Hargreaves and others, 1984).

While formal organizational features may help case management programs accomplish more standardizable tasks, they are not as well suited to those characterized by contingencies and unpredictability and may in fact interfere with performance in those areas. This issue underlies the recurrent debates regarding whether case management is a professional or paraprofessional role and whether the case manager should also be the client's primary therapist (Deitchman, 1980; Friday, 1986; Johnson and Rubin, 1983; Lamb, 1980; Levine, 1979; Rapp and Chamberlain, 1985).

One side argues that having a professional case manager–therapist is justified, even required, by the "special needs of long-term patients" (Lamb, 1980, p. 763)—needs better met through primary-group relations than bureaucratic ones (Deitchman, 1980):

The main problems facing the chronically disabled client in the community are economic and psychological survival. No one can "coordinate" survival. . . . For a chronic client to survive psychologically, he needs someone he can have a relationship with, someone he can confide in, someone he can depend on. . . . Chronic clients are lonely, isolated people whose greatest need is to learn the healing benefits that come from closeness to others [pp. 788–789].

Moreover, the unpredictability of both clients' lives and the tasks of case management are held to require a flexibility and responsiveness often lacking in the bureaucratic settings of paraprofessional case management, as provocatively portrayed in a commentary entitled "How Many Case Managers Does It Take to Screw in a Light Bulb?" (Deitchman, 1980).

On the other hand, those advocating use of paraprofessional case managers, separate from therapeutic functions, recognize the needs of mental health organizations and the service system as legitimate and critical determinants of the design of case management programs. They cite the inability of the service delivery system to afford professionals on the scale necessary for such programs (Rapp and Chamberlain, 1985) or to afford the professional philosophy of giving "the highest possible quality of care on a one-to-one basis to a limited number of clients" (Friday, 1986, p. 56).

Besides the advantages of cost and scale, arguments for paraprofessional case managers are bolstered by evidence that they are more able and willing than professionals to "work" the system for clients: They do more of the legwork necessary for service linkages and have more intimate knowledge of community service systems (Intagliata and Baker, 1983; Kurtz, Bagarozzi, and Pollane, 1984; Rapp and Chamberlain, 1985).

While the current expansion of paraprofessional case management programs is largely driven by economic and organizational factors, its exponents do not equate "the paraprofessional" with "the bureaucracy," as do its critics. To the contrary, paraprofessionals are held to be more focused on clients' everyday problems and more spontaneous in their reactions to them than professionals, whose therapeutic orientations can get in the way (Levine, 1979; Rapp and Chamberlain, 1985). In essence, the argument here is that paraprofessionals can combine the best features of both primary groups and formal organizations.

To date, this remains an issue characterized more by the heat of professional ideology than the illumination of systematic evaluation. There will continue to be a dialectic between the drive for more managerial approaches to case management and the need to provide the chronically mentally ill with a human ally with the skills and commitment to make the system work. Finding the best synthesis will require the talents of both professional therapists and paraprofessional case managers, and various combinations of the two roles have been developed or proposed (Lamb, 1980; Rapp and Chamberlain, 1985). The perspective presented here suggests that the future design of case management should be based primarily on an evaluation of its role in the organization of mental health and other human services, rather than on economic constraints or professional interests.

Conclusion

If the middle ground that case management occupies between formal organizations and primary groups offers great advantages, it creates, as well, a seemingly antithetical set of objectives: to provide a caretaker but also to promote clients' autonomy; to connect clients with services but to avoid socializing them to the role of chronic mental patient. To overcome this paradox requires flexibility, insight, and stamina on the part of the case manager, as well as training and supervisory structures that directly and supportively confront the uncomfortable ambiguities of the role.

As case management is disseminated through the mental health system and expanded to new service sectors, the proper balance between bureaucratic and primary-group qualities will become increasingly important. How much and how often can a role that claims as its domain the "whole person" be bureaucratized? How can client autonomy be protected, let alone enhanced, in such a system? Solutions to these and related issues must be sought if case management programs are to enable service systems and their clients, like formal organizations and primary groups, to perform most effectively in the presence of one another.

References

Aldrich, H., and Herker, D. "Boundary-Spanning Roles and Organization Structure." *Academy of Management Review*, 1977, 2, 217–230.
Altman, H. "Collaborative Discharge Planning for the Deinstitutionalized." *Social Work*, 1982, 27 (5), 422–427.
Baker, F., and Weiss, R. S. "The Nature of Case Management Support." *Hospital and Community Psychiatry*, 1984, 35 (9), 925–928.
Berzon, P., and Lowenstein, B. "A Flexible Model of Case Management." In B. Pepper, and H. Ryglewicz (eds.), *Advances in Treating the Young Adult Chronic Patient*. New Directions for Mental Health Services, no. 21. San Francisco: Jossey-Bass, 1984.
Caragonne, P. "An Analysis of the Function of the Case Manager in Four Mental Health Social Services Settings." Report of the Case Management Research Project. Austin: School of Social Work, University of Texas, 1980.
Cooley, C. H. *Social Organization*. New York: Scribner's, 1909.

Deitchman, W. S. "How Many Case Managers Does It Take to Screw in a Light Bulb?" *Hospital and Community Psychiatry,* 1980, *31* (11), 788–789.

Diamond, R. J., and Wikler, D. I. "Ethical Problems in Community Treatment of the Chronically Mentally Ill." In L. I. Stein, and M. A. Test (eds.), *The Training in Community Living Model: A Decade of Experience.* New Directions for Mental Health Services, no. 26. San Francisco: Jossey-Bass, 1985.

Friday, J. C. "Case Managers for the Chronically Mentally Ill: Assessing and Improving Their Performance." Atlanta: Southern Regional Education Board, 1986.

Goldstrom, I. D., and Manderscheid, R. W. "A Descriptive Analysis of Community Support Program Case Managers Serving the Chronically Mentally Ill." *Community Mental Health Journal,* 1983, *19* (1), 17–26.

Hargreaves, W. A., Shaw, R. E., Shadoan, R., Walker, E., Surber, R., and Gaynor, J. "Measuring Case Management Activity." *Journal of Nervous and Mental Disease,* 1984, *172* (5), 296–300.

Harris, M., and Bergman, H. C. "Case Management with the Chronically Mentally Ill: A Clinical Perspective." *American Journal of Orthopsychiatry,* 1987, *57* (2), 296–302.

Harrod, J. B. "Defining Case Management in Community Support Systems." *Psychosocial Rehabilitation Journal,* 1986, *9* (3), 56–61.

Intagliata, J. "Improving the Quality of Community Care for the Chronically Mentally Disabled: The Role of Case Management." *Schizophrenia Bulletin,* 1982, *8* (4), 655–674.

Intagliata, J., and Baker, F. "Factors Affecting Case Management Services for the Chronically Mentally Ill." *Administration in Mental Health,* 1983, *11* (2), 75–91.

Johnson, P. J., and Rubin, A. "Case Management in Mental Health: A Social Work Domain?" *Social Work,* 1983, *28* (1), 49–55.

Joint Commission on the Accreditation of Hospitals. *Principles for Accreditation of Community Mental Health Service Programs.* Chicago: Joint Commission on the Accreditation of Hospitals, 1976.

Kanter, J. S. "Case Management of the Young Adult Chronic Patient." In J. S. Kanter (ed.), *Clinical Issues in Treating the Chronic Mentally Ill.* New Directions for Mental Health Services, no. 27. San Francisco: Jossey-Bass, 1985.

Kemp, B. J. "The Case Management Model of Human Service Delivery." In E. L. Pan, T. E. Backer, and C. L. Vash (eds.), *Annual Review of Rehabilitation.* Vol. 2. New York: Springer, 1981.

Kurtz, L. F., Bagarozzi, D. A., and Pollane, L. P. "Case Management in Mental Health." *Health and Social Work,* 1984, *9* (3), 201–211.

Lamb, H. R. "Therapist–Case Managers: More than Brokers of Services." *Hospital and Community Psychiatry,* 1980, *31* (11), 762–764.

Levine, M. "Case Management: Lessons from Earlier Efforts." *Evaluation and Program Planning,* 1979, *2,* 235–243.

Levine, I. S., and Fleming, M. *Human Resource Development: Issues in Case Management.* Baltimore: Manpower Development Unit and Community Support Project, Maryland Mental Hygiene Administration, 1986.

Litwak, E. *Helping the Elderly: The Complementary Roles of Informal Networks and Formal Systems.* New York: Guilford Press, 1985.

Mechanic, D. "The Challenge of Chronic Mental Illness: A Retrospective and Prospective View." *Hospital and Community Psychiatry,* 1986, *37* (9), 891–896.

Minnesota Community Support Project. "Case Management." *The Minnesota Community Support Project Newsletter,* 1980, *3* (4), 1–10.

70

Mueller, B. J., and Hopp, M. "Attitudinal, Administrative, Legal, and Fiscal Barriers to Case Management in Social Rehabilitation of the Mentally Ill." *International Journal of Mental Health*, 1987, *15* (4), 44–58.

Platman, S. R., Dorgan, R. E., Gerhard, R. S., Mallam, K. E., and Spiliadis, S. S. "Case Management of the Mentally Disabled." *Journal of Public Health Policy*, 1982, *3* (3), 302–314.

Rapp, C. A., and Chamberlain, R. "Case Management Services for the Chronically Mentally Ill." *Social Work*, 1985, *30* (5), 417–422.

Schwartz, S. R., Goldman, H. H., and Churgin, S. "Case Management for the Chronically Mentally Ill: Models and Dimensions." *Hospital and Community Psychiatry*, 1982, *33* (12), 1006–1009.

Stroul, B. A. *Toward Community Support Systems for the Mentally Disabled: The NIMH Community Support Program.* Boston: Center for Rehabilitation, Research, and Training in Mental Health, Boston University, 1984.

Test, M. A. "Continuity of Care in Community Treatment." In L. I. Stein (ed.), *Community Support Systems for the Long-Term Patient.* New Directions for Mental Health Services, no. 2. San Francisco: Jossey-Bass, 1979.

Weber, M. *The Theory of Social Economic Organization.* (A. M. Henderson, and T. Parsons, eds. and trans.) New York: Oxford University Press, 1947.

Wolowitz, D. "Clients' Rights in a Case Management System." In C. J. Sanborn (ed.), *Case Management in Mental Health Services.* New York: Haworth Press, 1983.

Ann E. P. Dill is postdoctoral fellow in the Rutgers-Princeton Program in Mental Health Research at the Institute for Health, Health Care Policy, and Aging Research, Rutgers University.

*Statutory, organizational, and financial barriers in the
country's housing system, social resistance, and inadequate
service linkages must be addressed in order to provide the
chronically mentally ill with decent, affordable, and
appropriate housing.*

Obstacles in Urban Housing Policy for the Chronically Mentally Ill

Carol A. Boyer

Housing is a generic concern for all people but an especially difficult problem for the indigent chronically mentally ill (Ball and Havassy, 1984; Talbott, 1981; U.S. General Accounting Office, 1985). Their symptoms and impaired functioning make it difficult to acquire and keep housing, particularly in a highly competitive and extremely tight low-cost housing market. Their special needs require a sophisticated match of housing structures with social and rehabilitative services. With reduced federal involvement in the production, ownership, and management of housing, even more obstacles exist. Local conditions, as well, increasingly affect the availability of housing to the chronically mentally ill (CMI).

Background to the Housing Crisis for the CMI

Over the past few decades, a series of largely unrelated developments precipitated the current housing emergency for the CMI as well as for other low- and moderate-income groups. Between 1955 and 1984 the population of public mental hospitals decreased by almost 80 percent from 559,000 to 116,000 (Manderscheid, 1986). While the direct role of

D. Mechanic (ed.). *Improving Mental Health Services: What the Social Sciences Tell Us.*
New Directions for Mental Health Services, no. 36. San Francisco: Jossey-Bass, 1987.

deinstitutionalization of long-term patients on the problem of homelessness has been challenged, clearly many indigent mentally ill, especially younger adult chronics, have had difficulty staying housed. Most long-term patients who were discharged went to their families or to nursing homes, but a smaller proportion, living in board-and-care homes and single-room occupancy hotels, were the most vulnerable to homelessness (Bassuk and Lamb, 1986). Most surveys show that one-third of the homeless have been hospitalized in a psychiatric facility; the median age of this group is thirty-four to forty years (Bassuk and Lamb, 1986; New York State Office of Mental Health, 1982; Rossi, Fisher, and Willis, 1986; Roth, Bean, Lust, and Saveanu, 1985). These studies reveal that the bulk of the homeless population has *not* had prior state hospitalization, nor have these people typically been discharged from the hospital to the street. Most of the homeless mentally ill are young adult chronics who have never been hospitalized or who have had recurrent short hospital stays.

Sufficient housing and other social and therapeutic support services have not been mobilized to serve either the long-term deinstitutionalized patients or the young adult chronics. Less than 800 of the originally planned 2,000 community mental health centers (CMHCs) were established nationally (National Institute of Mental Health, 1980). Even within those existing CMHCs, resources were often targeted to less severely ill individuals. While the federal Community Support Program (CSP) was implemented in 1977 to respond to the failures of deinstitutionalization and CMHCs, it has been a modestly funded program only capable of helping a small fraction of the homeless CMI.

Attempts to avoid long-term hospital stays through "admission diversion policies" have compounded housing problems for the CMI (Talbott and Lamb, 1984). When chronic mental patients suffer from an exacerbation of their symptoms, they are not readily admitted to state hospitals. Alternatively, they may have brief hospital stays and be discharged without stable living arrangements. Moreover, some of the homeless CMI resist what support is available for housing and other social services.

Economic problems widen these gaps in the functioning of the mental health system. With the passage of the Omnibus Budget Reconciliation Act of 1981, eligibility standards for the Social Security Disability Insurance (SSDI) program were tightened, and the rate of growth of other social welfare programs benefiting the CMI decreased. These social welfare spending cuts were accompanied by previous wider system changes, including economic stagnation, high employment levels, rising inflation, and declining real wages. All of these economic factors reduced the ability of the CMI to find and maintain decent, affordable, and appropriate housing.

Several aspects of the low-cost housing crisis have affected the availability and accessibility of housing for the CMI: First, with the median gross rent as a percentage of median income rising from 22 percent to 29 percent between 1973 and 1981, it became increasingly difficult for the indigent CMI to find affordable housing. In fact, for renters with $3,000 or less annual income, a group that includes many CMI, the median rent-income ratio was more than 60 percent (U.S. Bureau of the Census, 1983). Rossi and Wright (1987), studying the homeless in Chicago, described them as "the poorest of the poor, surviving on less than 40 percent of a poverty-level income" (p. 100).

Second, forced displacement as a result of rent increases, conversion of rental units to condominiums, fire, redevelopment, and under-maintenance were more likely to affect the indigent, including most CMI (Hartman, Keating, and LeGates, 1982).

Third, cheap housing has virtually disappeared. It is far more difficult than before for the CMI to find inexpensive rooms in hotels, in other single-room occupancies, or in apartments. Rental vacancy rates are low in many large cities (such as Philadelphia, Baltimore, and Cincinnati) and their standard metropolitan statistical areas (SMSAs) (Philadelphia, 4 percent; Baltimore, 5.2 percent; Cincinnati, 4-5 percent; Columbus, 5-6 percent), and housing is even scarcer in New York, San Francisco, and Boston with ranges between 1 and 2 percent (Hopper and Hamberg, 1986; U.S. Bureau of the Census, 1985; Van Meter, 1986). Yet, even where vacancy rates are higher, such as in Austin (16.1 percent) and Charlotte (9.3 percent), many CMI remain homeless (Aiken, Somers, and Shore, 1986; Van Meter, 1986); the availability of housing alone does not result in living space for the CMI.

Each of these factors contributed to the current housing problems for the CMI. Strategies to overcome these problems can be formulated only if we understand the complex obstacles that specifically stand in the way of adequate housing for the CMI.

The Housing Needs of the CMI

To understand and address the existing obstacles to urban housing for the CMI, I shall first describe the conditions necessary for appropriately housing the CMI. Ideally, one would expect to achieve the following standards, although few attempts have been made to test the elements critical to the housing environment for the CMI (Allard and others, 1986; Paterson and Rhubright, 1986):

- Safe, affordable, decent low-income or subsidized housing with stable financing
- A "residential continuum" to meet varying functional capacities of the CMI and to encourage movement toward independent living

- A site convenient to support services and public transportation
- Linkage to a range of therapeutic and social services, including crisis intervention, case management, vocational rehabilitation, and socialization programs
- Integration of the CMI into neighborhood and community life
- Legal safeguards protecting against exclusionary zoning ordinances and unwarranted dislocation
- Interagency cooperation in optimizing housing, therapeutic, and social services.

A Typology of Obstacles

In the following subsections, I propose five types of obstacles to meeting these goals. These obstacles include explicit actions by policy makers, agency personnel, and communities to limit housing options for the homeless CMI. Less visible but no less critical may be unstated assumptions that detour the implementation of housing policies and mitigate against the CMI getting the housing that they need.

Statutory Obstacles. This category includes the absence of legislation to facilitate access to housing for the CMI and to protect them from housing discrimination. The CMI need special protections in their search for housing. Their "consumption disability," coupled with a tight housing market, limits their ability to find housing and prompts landlords to refuse to rent to them (Rossi, Fisher, and Willis, 1986). Local zoning regulations and restrictive covenants have barred the establishment of group homes and comprised the rights of the mentally ill to locate in many neighborhoods.

Housing has not been viewed as a social right in the United States, nor is housing welfare for the poor vigorously supported by positive government action. The landmark Housing Act of 1949 adopted more of a "social service philosophy" than a legal mandate in setting the national goal of "a decent home in a suitable living environment for all Americans" (Lundqvist, 1986, p. 31). Though rights to shelter and housing are recognized in several states and cities, many problems concerning the extent of public obligations remain. The Overnight Shelter Act (Initiative 17), approved by referendum in the District of Columbia in 1984, highlights some outstanding issues. The act has been challenged by city officials because of the costs of implementing the shelter bill. The act may also be overturned because the city charter prohibits a referendum to obligate spending from district coffers. Other criticisms of the act concern its prohibition on sheltering homeless from neighboring states and the fact that the services offered do not include rehabilitative and other social therapies.

Equally problematic are government statutes in regulating residential facilities for the CMI. Bardach (1977) examined the illusory benefits of licensing board-and-care facilities for the mentally ill in California and concluded that licensing does not result in the upgrading of facilities, that standards are limited to "bricks and mortar," that denial and revocation of licenses are generally impossible, and that threats of revocation do not improve care.

Organizational annd Administrative Obstacles. These obstacles are located both within the agencies responsible for planning and providing services and in the relationships between them. Broad areas of uncertainty exist about the implementation of housing plans for the CMI, including agency struggles about policy goals, poor coordination, duplication of efforts, territorial disputes, and insufficient backup services. A mix of fragmented social and rehabilitative services often fails to support what stable living arrangements may have been found.

No single federal program supports the range of clinical and social services needed for the CMI. With multiple agencies and multiple actors pursuing their own special interests and goals, the classic "implementation problem" has arisen (Bardach, 1977), creating major problems in management and in the service delivery capacity of those organizations. Some of these organizational limitations were highlighted in a congressionally mandated report by the U.S. Departments of Health and Human Services (HHS) and Housing and Urban Development (HUD) (1983). The joint report concluded that the federal initiatives for the homeless in "most HHS programs were not designed with their unique needs in mind" (p. 18). Moreover, HUD programs "were developed to serve a much broader population" (p. 22) without resources tailored to the needs of the CMI.

Several of the nation's largest cities are now developing centralized mental health authorities under a demonstration project jointly sponsored by the Robert Wood Johnson Foundation, HUD, and several agencies in HHS (Aiken, Somers, and Shore, 1986). Under these authorities, efforts will be made to integrate clinical, social (including housing), organizational, and fiscal responsibilities. Experts from private-sector housing development are assisting each of the cities with planning, construction, management, and marketing. Still, the complex organizational histories of the major agencies involved in caring for the CMI, as well as professional turf battles and political conflicts, will not be quickly or easily reversed.

Financial Obstacles. These obstacles are an obvious source of housing policy failure. Inadequate funding diminishes both the availability and quality of shelter and housing. In many states and localities, major financial resources in the mental health system remain tied to state mental institutions, not to community-based services. Financial difficulties, however, extend beyond the scarcity of funds. Federal monies appropriated through the Federal Emergency Management Agency (FEMA) and its Emergency Food and Shelter National Board Program carry severe restrictions on use, including a strict prohibition against capital expenditures and direct personnel costs.

Probably the most serious financial issues concern HUD's continuing budget cuts and the agency's increasing reliance on direct subsidies to tenants through Section 8 certificates and the newer voucher system, rather than on public housing or construction financing. According to Hartman (1986a), "the government is mounting a massive retreat from the housing role it began to assume during the New Deal" (p. 76). Its retreat is recognized in the cancellation of housing programs, in the lowering of the quality of housing supported under HUD programs, and in the drastic cuts in long-run budgetary commitments to housing, notably a 40 percent reduction between 1980 and 1985 (Executive Office of the President, 1985). Certificates and vouchers also fit the HUD's stance that no housing shortage exists in the United States, that the major problem is affordability. Affordability is hardly the only problem for the CMI.

Certificates and vouchers are not an ideal subsidy for the CMI. First, these tenant-based subsidies are limited, especially subsidies targeted to the CMI. Generally, other needy groups have a higher priority when local public housing authorities dispense them.

Second, their usability is compromised by the lack of decent, moderately priced vacant units, discrimination by owners, and a mismatch of vacant units to needs (Hartman, 1986b). HUD estimates that each year one-quarter of all available certificates and vouchers are not used (Riordan, 1987). For the 1980–1982 period, 36 percent of New York City residents issued certificates were unable to use them (Hartman, 1986b).

Third, the CMI do not benefit from the purported advantages of these subsidies—namely, the freedom of choice in selecting housing that certificates allow tenants and the support for private-sector development.

Fourth, little flexibility exists in the use of these subsidies. They cannot be attached to specific structures that might be operated by mental health authorities. Thus, a potential source of stable subsidization for housing that might offer rehabilitative and other support services cannot be realized. Additionally, certificates and vouchers cannot be used to keep their holders from moving, nor can they be used in temporary shelters.

Thus, substantial ambiguity and complexity arise in the use and management of these certificates and vouchers for the CMI. Success will depend on the "enabling" context in which the subsidies are used: Will housing stock be available? Will landlords rent to the CMI? Will neighborhoods accept the residential placement of the CMI?

Mortgage lenders and other providers of housing credit, such as bankers, state housing finance agencies, and private foundations, see local mental health service systems as being high financial risks (Carling,

1980). Funding for construction or rehabilitation requires collateral, a strong credit history, a commitment to providing support services, and plans to locate the residence for the CMI in a stable environment—a set of conditions that most mental health agencies cannot meet.

Housing Market and Residential-Specific Obstacles. This category refers to a range of housing resource scarcities and the inadequacy of social and therapeutic services linked to housing. Wright and Lam (1987) report that the number of low-income rental housing units for twelve large American cities declined by 30 percent from the late 1970s to the early 1980s. In New York alone, the 53,000 single-room occupancy units in 1979 declined to 15,000 in 1984 (U.S. Department of Health and Human Services, 1984). Condominium conversion, gentrification, abandonment, demolition, "disinvestment," and arson considerably reduced available housing for the CMI (Brady, 1983; Hartman, Keating, and LeGates, 1982).

Direct federal supply of housing for the homeless has failed to produce the number of anticipated units. For fiscal year 1984, the U.S. Department of Defense (DOD) received $8 million from Congress for the renovation of vacant military facilities for use as emergency shelters. The DOD identified 600 potential sites, but only two facilities were renovated for $900,000. Resistance to opening the shelters was encountered from local politicians, residents, and military base commanders.

Through an agreement with the Federal Task Force for the Homeless, the General Services Administration promised a number of its 3,874 surplus federal buildings for use as emergency shelters, but only three buildings were eventually offered. HUD also agreed to offer some of the agency's 9,225 unsold properties as single-family homes. Only ten homes were provided, all of them in Memphis, Tennessee (Committee on Government Operations, 1985). Thus, even when a potential supply of housing exists, a host of obstacles (organizational, administrative, social resistance, and others) undermine availability and access for the CMI.

Not to be underestimated is the potential rejection of available housing options by the CMI themselves, although the extent of this problem has not been empirically examined. Also, adequate services to assist the mentally ill, as well as experienced operators and landlords who can serve the CMI, may be lacking in available residences and reduce the "survival" of the CMI in such housing.

Social Resistance. Public attitudes about the mentally ill—intolerance, prejudice, stigmatization, and abhorrence—are translated into social resistance, the last obstacle to be discussed. Opposition to housing the CMI in neighborhoods focuses on such issues as the decline of property values, the delay of revitalization efforts, and threats to public safety ("Residents Fight Plan . . . ," 1986). Research on neighborhood housing of the mentally retarded does not show these negative effects. Wolpert

(1978) and Dolan and Wolpert (1982), for example, showed that group homes for mentally retarded persons generated no greater property value declines or higher turnover rates than matched controls. Still, neighborhoods typically prefer alternative uses for available housing—even drug rehabilitation.

Public resistance may occur at a number of stages in the development of housing for the CMI. Local opposition can block the initial application for housing. Backdoor approaches to opening group homes frequently backfire and may stir high neighborhood resentment. Petitions express citizen rejection of shelter and housing for the CMI once established, usually claiming dangerous and unreasonable behavior, inadequate maintenance, and loitering. Citizen protest may also prevent renewal of the lease. Typically, upper-middle-class neighbors offer greater opposition to group homes than do other socioeconomic groups (Hogan, 1986).

The success of inducements for homeowners and renters to accept group homes, either for transitional or for long-term housing, has not been studied. Tax remissions might limit social resistance, although the implication might be that home values will decrease if the CMI move in. A calculation of "fair share," where neighborhoods accept some responsibility for housing, could avoid oversaturation, but how would communities respond to this attempt at social justice?

Community resistance is not easily overcome. Its sources range from ignorance, confusion, and indifference to fear and anger. Public education campaigns and collaborative working groups of advocates, public officials, and neighborhoods may ease the struggle, but considerable readjustments will be required before community-based residences for the CMI are a more common feature in the city landscape.

Conclusion

Long-term solutions for housing the CMI necessitate overcoming tenacious and complex obstacles. Yet, enthusiastic, inspiring, and creative endeavors are now seen in many areas. Communities and their local mental health and housing authorities have realized the importance of housing in the continuum of services for the CMI. Interagency agreements for maintaining social welfare and housing subsidies have been adopted for clients admitted temporarily to hospitals and community programs. Formal site-selection procedures involving neighborhoods, residence operators, and local municipalities have been established. HUD has targeted Section 8 certificates for the CMI in a national demonstration program. Medicaid waivers offer an additional resource base for outpatient and community-based care. A few states have redirected state funds from hospitals to community programs.

On the other hand, inequities in housing policy and inefficiencies in implementing government programs for housing remain. Sustaining the new and creative endeavors, extending them nationally, and addressing the host of other obstacles will be critical to meeting the housing needs of the CMI.

References

Aiken, L. H., Somers, S., and Shore, M. F. "Private Foundations in Health Affairs: A Case Study of the Development of a National Initiative for the Chronically Mentally Ill." *American Psychologist*, 1986, *41*, 1290-1295.

Allard, M. A., Carling, P. J., Bradley, V., Spence, R., Randolph, F., and Ridgway, P. "Providing Housing and Supports for People with Psychiatric Disabilities: A Technical Assistance Manual for Applicants for the Robert Wood Johnson Foundation and U.S. Department of Housing and Urban Development Program for the 'Chronically Mentally Ill.'" Rockville, Md.: National Institute of Mental Health, 1986.

Ball, F.L.J., and Havassy, B. E. "A Survey of the Problems and Needs of Homeless Consumers of Acute Psychiatric Services." *Hospital and Community Psychiatry*, 1984, *35*, 917-921.

Bardach, E. *The Implementation Game*. Cambridge: Massachusetts Institute of Technology Press, 1977.

Bassuk, E. L., and Lamb, H. R. "Homelessness and the Implementation of Deinstitutionalization." In E. L. Bassuk (ed.), *The Mental Health Needs of Homeless Persons*. New Directions for Mental Health Services, no. 30. San Francisco: Jossey-Bass, 1986.

Brady, J. "Arson, Urban Economy, and Organized Crime: The Case of Boston." *Social Problems*, 1983, *31*, 1-27.

Carling, P. J. "Choreography with an Uncertain Score: Federal Collaboration in Housing and Mental Health." Rockville, Md.: National Institute of Mental Health, 1980.

Committee on Government Operations. "The Federal Response to the Homeless Crisis." Washington, D.C.: U.S. Government Printing Office, 1985.

Dolan, L. W., and Wolpert, J. "Long-Term Neighborhood Property Impacts of Group Homes for Mentally Retarded People." Woodrow Wilson School Discussion Paper Series, Princeton: Princeton University, 1982.

Executive Office of the President. *Budget of the United States Government, Fiscal Year 1987*. Washington, D.C.: U.S. Government Printing Office, 1985.

Hartman, C. "The Housing Part of the Homelessness Problem." In E. L. Bassuk (ed.), *The Mental Health Needs of Homeless Persons*. New Directions for Mental Health Services, no. 30. San Francisco: Jossey-Bass, 1986a.

Hartman, C. "Housing Policies Under the Reagan Administration." In R. G. Bratt, C. Hartman, and A. Meyerson (eds.), *Critical Perspectives on Housing*. Philadelphia: Temple University Press, 1986b.

Hartman, C., Keating, D., and LeGates, R. *Displacement: How to Fight It*. Berkeley: National Housing Law Project, 1982.

Hogan, R. "Community Opposition to Group Homes." *Social Science Quarterly*, 1986, *67*, 442-449.

Hopper, K., and Hamberg, J. "The Making of America's Homeless: From Skid Row to New Poor, 1945-1984." In R. G. Bratt, C. Hartman, and A. Meyerson (eds.), *Critical Perspectives on Housing*. Philadelphia: Temple University Press, 1986.

Lundqvist, L. J. *Housing Policy and Equality.* Dover, N.H.: Croom Helm, 1986.

Manderscheid, R. W. Personal communication. Washington, D.C.: Survey and Reports Branch, Division of Biometry and Applied Science, National Institute of Mental Health, 1986.

Marin, P. "Helping and Hating the Homeless." *Harper's,* 1987, *274,* 39–49.

National Institute of Mental Health. *History of the Community Mental Health Centers Program.* Rockville, Md.: National Institute of Mental Health, 1980.

New York State Office of Mental Health. *Who Are the Homeless? A Study of Randomly Selected Men Who Use New York City Shelters.* New York: New York State Office of Mental Health, 1982.

Paterson, A., and Rhubright, E. "Housing for the Mentally Ill: A Place Called Home." In *State Legislative Report.* Vol. 11, no. 9. Denver: National Conference of State Legislatures, 1986.

"Residents Fight Plan for Staten Island's First City Shelter for Homeless." *New York Times,* August 28, 1986, p. B1.

Riordan, T. "Housekeeping at HUD." *Common Cause,* 1987, *13,* 26–31.

Rossi, P. H., Fisher, G. A., and Willis, G. *The Condition of the Homeless of Chicago.* Amherst: Social and Demographic Research Institute, University of Massachusetts, 1986.

Rossi, P. H., and Wright, J. D. "The Determinants of Homelessness." *Health Affairs,* 1987, *6,* 19–32.

Roth, D., Bean, J., Lust, N., and Saveanu, T. *Homelessness in Ohio: A Study of People in Need.* Columbus: Ohio Department of Mental Health, 1985.

Talbott, J. A. "The National Plan for the Chronically Mentally Ill: A Programmatic Analysis." *Hospital and Community Psychiatry,* 1981, *32,* 699–704.

Talbott, J. A., and Lamb, H. R. "Summary and Recommendations." In H. R. Lamb (ed.), *The Homeless Mentally Ill: A Task Force Report of the American Psychiatric Association.* Washington, D.C.: American Psychiatric Association, 1984.

U.S. Bureau of the Census. *Annual Housing Survey, Part C: Financial Characteristics of the Housing Inventory.* Washington, D.C.: U.S. Government Printing Office, 1983.

U.S. Bureau of the Census. *Census of Population and Housing Estimates of Social, Economic, and Housing Characteristics for States and Selected SMSAs.* Washington, D.C.: U.S. Government Printing Office, 1985.

U.S. Department of Health and Human Services. *The Homeless: Background, Analysis, and Options.* Washington, D.C.: U.S. Department of Health and Human Services, 1984.

U.S. Departments of Health and Human Services and Housing and Urban Development. *Report on Federal Efforts to Respond to the Shelter and Basic Living Needs of Chronically Mentally Ill Individuals.* Washington, D.C.: U.S. Government Printing Office, 1983.

U.S. General Accounting Office. *Homelessness: A Complex Problem and the Federal Response.* Washington, D.C.: U.S. General Accounting Office, 1985.

Van Meter, E. Personal communication. Washington, D.C.: Office of Policy Development and Research, U.S. Department of Housing and Urban Development, 1986.

Wolpert, J. "Group Homes for the Mentally Retarded: An Investigation of Neighborhood Property Impacts." Unpublished manuscript, Princeton University, 1978.

Wright, J. D., and Lam, J. "The Low-Income Housing Supply and the Problem of Homelessness." *Social Policy,* 1987, *17* (4), 48–53.

Carol A. Boyer is postdoctoral fellow in the Rutgers-Princeton Program in Mental Health Research at the Institute for Health, Health Care Policy, and Aging Research, Rutgers University.

To avoid reinstitutionalization of judgment-impaired
individuals, community mental health needs to build its
capacity for serving uncooperative persons who face high risks
of physical or environmental harm.

Substituted Judgment
and Protective Intervention

Stephen Crystal, Edmund Dejowski

Substantial numbers of persons in the population suffer from mental impairments that compromise their ability to meet the basic needs of life or to make decisions affecting their everyday well-being or safety. This can be the result of mental illness or of other conditions, such as mental retardation, substance abuse, or the organic dementias of old age.

Most persons with these conditions are able to manage their daily affairs with little or no help. But functional or judgmental impairment can bring with it increased risk—typically to the safety or well-being of the impaired individual, but not infrequently to others as well.

Many impaired persons who face endangering situations fail to recognize the danger, do not know help is available, do not want help, or misunderstand or mistrust potential helpers. For these and other reasons, judgment-impaired persons at risk are usually not served until the emergence of a severe threat to life or health. Typical precipitating events include gross sanitation or fire hazards in living quarters; lack of heat, imminent eviction; unpaid utility or other bills; apparent malnutrition or untreated physical illness; homelessness; wandering; and hospitalization of individuals believed to be unable to return home safely.

D. Mechanic (ed.). *Improving Mental Health Services: What the Social Sciences Can Tell Us.*
New Directions for Mental Health Services, no. 36. San Francisco: Jossey-Bass, 1987.

The Protective Role

In an earlier era, individuals who behaved bizarrely and whose ability to look after their own needs was in doubt were likely to be institutionalized. With the recent swing away from such reliance, the threshold for civil commitment has been substantially (and properly) raised. These developments, however, have created a need for community-based systems for monitoring risk and for protective intervention. As many communities discovered later than they should have, appropriate implementation of deinstitutionalization calls for the development of a range of noninstitutional mechanisms for patient management. Mental health providers need to take an increasingly active role in implementing these services.

The failure of community mental health to fill the protective function that was served by civil commitment for disorganized, noncompliant persons is only one factor contributing to the sad neglect of mentally ill people that can be documented on the streets of any city in the country. Nonetheless, the failure of the community mental health care system to protect the mentally ill is being cited by some as an indicator that deinstitutionalization has gone too far. If the mental health system continues to neglect this protective function, many of the chronically mentally ill may continue to face unacceptable risks, and pressures for reinstitutionalization will grow.

There are, however, obstacles to the development of a more proactive role by community mental health providers. For example, many remain deeply committed to the principle that mental health services can and should be provided only to those who want them. The model of a client voluntarily meeting scheduled appointments in a clinic has remained widespread in community mental health practice despite a recognition by many that the most disturbed persons could not be expected to function in such an orderly and compliant way.

The protective role requires serving many who are adamantly opposed to assistance of any kind. Some traditional modes of mental health treatment—such as psychotherapy, day programs, and even medication clinics—will be unavailing for most of these persons. For the resistant yet at-risk population, the need instead is for service systems that can reach out to identify and evaluate dangerous conditions, reduce risks, and monitor apparently stabilized situations.

Those Potentially At Risk

The number of individuals *potentially* at risk is substantial. The frail elderly suffering from the dementias of old age are the largest group and the "core constituency" for adult protective services programs (Hall and Mathiasen, 1973). Pooling data from several epidemiological studies, Kay and Bergmann (1980) have estimated the prevalence of organic brain syndromes among persons over sixty-five at 6.3 percent and among those over eighty at 17.7 percent; of these, 75 percent were living in the community. The prevalence of moderate to profound mental retardation has been estimated at 0.2 percent of the general population, representing about 350,000 adult individuals (American Psychiatric Association, 1980). Estimates of the prevalence of schizophrenia vary depending on the breadth of diagnostic criteria applied and other factors. U.S. lifetime prevalence estimates tend to be in the 1 to 2 percent range (American Psychiatric Association, 1980), and a point prevalence of 0.5 percent would be well within the range of published estimates, translating to about 900,000 persons. Only about 125,000 individuals of all diagnoses combined reside at a given time in public psychiatric hospitals (Mechanic, 1986), suggesting that only a rather small percentage of schizophrenic individuals are hospitalized at any given time.

Thus, without including many other categories of individuals, such as substance abusers and the severely mentally ill other than schizophrenics, the estimates for these three risk categories represent something on the order of three million adults who *may* periodically or chronically be substantially impaired in judgment and endangered as a result. Some reside in institutions, but the majority are in the community; of those in the community, a relatively small proportion live in protected settings such as group residences, others live with family members able and willing to look after them, but a large number lack such support. The largest group of at-risk persons, the very old, tend to have outlived spouses (and often family) and are living alone in larger numbers as part of a general tendency to independent living on the part of the elderly. Altogether there are several hundred thousand individuals with severely compromised mental or judgmental capacity living alone in the community, who are likely to be at risk.

Potential risk does not, of course, mean that intervention by mental health professionals is required, but it does indicate the kind of population that should be targeted for particular attention by the community mental provider in fulfilling the protective function of community care. The numbers of potentially at-risk persons, while not uncountable or unmanageable, are larger than generally presumed, and they represent groups such as the elderly that are historically underserved by community mental health programs (Flemming, Buchanan, Santos, and Rickards, 1984).

Risk Assessment

People take risks all the time. Parachutists, smokers, and subway riders endure risks that some would regard as unacceptably high. Our respect for an individual's right to make even disastrous personal choices dictates against meddling with such behavior. Persons with impaired judgment may, like anyone else, choose to take risks. The uninvited involvement of mental health professionals becomes appropriate when the choice to endure the risky behavior is related to the impairment of judgment—for example, when a delusion directs a person to commit a dangerous act. As the relationship between the impairment and the risky behavior becomes less direct, the appropriateness of intervention becomes less clear. Examples include circumstances in which impaired judgment simply interferes with the capacity to recognize or appreciate the risks entailed in certain behavior or to recognize personal limitations that make some common situations unreasonably risky. Under such circumstances, the decision to intervene should be based on weighing both the degree of risk and the degree of impairment.

Identification of risk factors is a vital function in protecting endangered adults. The assessment of risk can entail the same diagnostic, intelligence, and behavioral assessments that mental health providers customarily perform. But often service choices must be made on short notice with little information about the client, in the face of an active refusal to cooperate, and usually with an imminent catastrophe at hand. These conditions will require a departure from standard diagnostic practice. Standardized methods and instruments appropriate to many of these circumstances are available and can improve accuracy, as well as credibility, if the professional judgment made during a crisis is later challenged (Daiches, 1983). The professional should be acquainted with measures of physical functioning, to determine impairments in daily living activities (Katz and others, 1963), and measures of social support, such as the Network Analysis Profile (Sokolovsky and Cohen, 1981). The major multidimensional measures have been reviewed by Kane and Kane (1981). A functional assessment tool has also been developed to determine the need for guardianship (Saunders and Simon, 1987). A standard system for assessing the need for protection has also gained some acceptance. Adaptations of the Assessment for Protective Services, developed under a federally funded national demonstration project (Crystal, Dejowski, Flemming, and Daiches, 1982), are now included in administrative directives to local protective agencies in several states. In addition, assessments of the need for protection can be made more comprehensive if they are conducted by a team representing several disciplines (Regan, 1978; Schogt and Sadavoy, 1987).

Assuming Responsibility for the Person At Risk

Many endangered individuals fall between bureaucratic cracks, with no provider being willing to take primary responsibility for ongoing management. Mental health and other service professionals often regard such persons as the responsibility of local departments of social services through the adult protective services (APS) agency. However, as a national study of such agencies found, the designated APS agency nearly always has a very limited legislative and regulatory mandate and is typically allowed to intervene only during a present or imminent life threat. Very often, mental health providers refer at-risk clients to an APS agency and are very dissatisfied with the result. The APS worker, on the other hand, often states that mental health workers don't understand the role of APS and try to "dump" difficult clients for whom the mental health professional should provide continuing care (Crystal, Dejowski, Flemming, and Daiches, 1982). The long-term management of persons at risk can almost never be provided by the APS agency after the crisis has stabilized.

The mental health provider needs to understand the functions of the adult protective services agency. With some judgment-impaired clients, the public agency will be an appropriate source of referral and assistance. For most at-risk individuals, APS will not be available. The mental health provider cannot usually rely on referral to external sources to meet the protective needs of endangered, judgment-impaired persons.

Goals of Risk Management

Theorists and practitioners alike often subscribe to the mutually contradictory goals of reducing endangerment on the one hand and preserving independent self-direction on the other (Hall and Mathiasen, 1973; Blenkner, Bloom, Neilsen, and Webber, 1974). The result is a chronic tension in the practitioner's role between "authoritative" and "persuasive" methods of service. These terms are used to refer respectively to services that override the stated or implied wishes of the client, and to those in which the client remains the ultimate arbiter in decisions about how and where he or she will live. Work with any one client may involve a mix of both approaches. Little or no evidence is available regarding the relative effectiveness of either approach. But greater amounts of intervention may actually increase risk for some clients (Blenkner, Bloom, and Neilsen, and Webber, 1974). The generally acknowledged principle is to apply the least intervention that will suffice to protect the individual from serious and foreseeable harm. The goal is not to eliminate the risks of life; it is to identify and help alleviate those imminent and severe risks that result from judgmental impairment.

Tools for the Management of Risk

Most endangered persons can be served through aggressive, persistent, persuasive approaches, and regular monitoring. Some mental health programs serving endangered adults resistant to service, such as outreach programs for the mentally ill homeless who reject shelters, utilize noncoercive approaches with considerable success (Cohen, Putnam, and Sullivan, 1984). Nonetheless, there is general agreement among those serving such clients that involuntary intervention is sometimes essential to prevent serious harm (Regan and Springer, 1977).

One mechanism for involuntary intervention is guardianship, a status mediated by a court, whereby one individual makes decisions that are legally binding on another. All states have some form of guardianship. Some, such as California, have a special form of guardianship designed for the chronically mentally ill; others, like New York, have special guardianships for the developmentally disabled or mentally retarded.

But the usefulness of guardianship in its current forms in protecting the person with impaired judgment is limited. An endangered person with impaired judgment may not reach the legal threshold for involuntary intervention, or sufficient evidence may not be available to demonstrate the degree of impairment. Furthermore, one's status changes over time, and guardianship is not adaptable to the circumstances of persons who fluctuate in capacity, since a guardian should be discharged whenever the individual regains capacity. Usually the proceedings take far too long for guardianship to offer the solution to a present crisis.

Finding a person to serve as guardian for moderate- and low-income clients is also problematic. Court-designated guardians are often attorneys not anxious to take non-fee-generating cases and not sufficiently knowledgeable about community care to arrange the necessary services. The consequence is the overuse of nursing homes by many guardians. Public guardian programs exist in many places but are often fraught with problems such as unreasonably large caseloads and eligibility restrictions (Schmidt, Miller, Bell, and New, 1979).

Sometimes public guardian functions are filled by entities that have serious conflicts of interest in that role. For example, public social service agencies often serve as guardian for persons for whom they must make entitlement eligibility determinations. As a public official, a local or state social services commissioner must take a prudent approach to making determinations of public liability for applicants for assistance. As guardian, however, the commissioner should advocate for the broadest interpretation of the ward's eligibility for benefits and services. The viewpoints are unlikely to be identical, and it is equally unlikely that the commissioner would sue himself or herself to achieve resolution. Furthermore, the traditionally personal relationship between guardian and ward may be impaired if a public agency acts as guardian (Axilbund, 1981).

A 1972 report (Alexander and Lewin) documented that guardianship laws are frequently invoked without protecting adequately the due-process rights of the allegedly endangered person. These researchers found that the authority of the substitute decision maker is often abused.

Legislative advocacy and law reform over the ensuing decade have not fully alleviated these problems (Peters, Schmidt, and Miller, 1985). Even though legislative reform has resulted in creating more flexible forms of guardianship in many states, some believe that the inadequacy of available community services and public benefits will vitiate any legislative reform (Axilbund, 1981).

While some continue to favor the further revision of guardian laws, several alternatives appear more promising for filling the protective void left by deinstitutionalization, while allowing the client to retain greater personal independence. For many persons at risk, the only intervention required will be the management of a Social Security Income or Social Security Disability Income check. If evidence can establish a history of mismanagement and a condition likely to result in future mismanagement, the Social Security Administration can designate a representative payee to receive the checks and manage the funds for the beneficiary. This is an administrative process requiring no court involvement. Some community mental health agencies have established representative payee programs for their at-risk clients, with the agency serving as payee (Crystal, Dejowski, Flemming, and Daiches, 1982).

When, during crises, immediate legal authority for intervention is required, the provider may petition a court for a protective order. Such an order may authorize specific interventions, such as the provision of involuntary health care or other services, or temporary removal of the client from a dangerous environment. Specific legislation is unnecessary to enable courts to issue such orders, but, because of the reluctance of many courts to use their equitable powers to restrict personal liberty, several states have adopted legislation specifically authorizing short-term protective orders for endangered persons (for example, New York's Social Services Law, Section 473(b)). Such laws may create no new powers. However, they serve to display legislative intent that the power be exercised, and they may expand the procedural rights of the respondents, thereby increasing the willingness of many courts to issue orders. A study tracking the use of such legislation in New York City from its passage in 1981 through 1984 indicates a judicious and modest usage of the power, with under thirty applications citywide over three years (New York City Human Resources Administration, 1984).

Finally, remedies akin to civil commitment but aimed at community care are gaining renewed interest. Community commitment, which does not require hospitalization as a precedent condition, is the subject of experimentation in several states (Mulvey, Geller, and Roth, 1987) and is discussed in this sourcebook in Chapter Ten. Such remedies may offer the authority required to provide essential risk-reducing services and may also serve to channel the necessary funding to community mental health services so that they can fulfill adequately their protective functions.

90

Community mental health providers have not adequately responded to the protective needs of the judgment-impaired. The coercive aspects of protection are, for many providers, inconsistent with their professional role. Nonetheless, the reduction in census of the mental hospitals as well as other sociodemographic and economic changes have left a void in the care of the judgment-impaired that community mental health providers are now challenged to fill.

References

Alexander, G. J., and Lewin, T.H.D. *The Aged and the Need for Surrogate Management.* Syracuse, N.Y.: Syracuse University Press, 1972.

American Psychiatric Association. *Diagnostic and Statistical Manual of Mental Disorders.* (3rd ed.) Washington, D.C.: American Psychiatric Association, 1980.

Axilbund, M. T. *Exercising Judgment for the Disabled: Executive Summary.* Washington, D.C.: American Bar Association Commission on the Mentally Disabled, 1981.

Blenkner, M., Bloom, M., Neilsen, M., and Webber, R. *Final Report—Protective Services for Older People: Findings from the Benjamin Rose Institute Study.* Cleveland, Ohio: Benjamin Rose Institute, 1974.

Cohen, N. L., Putnam, J. E., and Sullivan, A. M. "The Mentally Ill Homeless: Isolation and Adaptation." *Hospital and Community Psychiatry,* 1984, *35,* 922–924.

Crystal, S., Dejowski, E., Flemming, C., and Daiches, S. *Adult Protective Services: The State of the Art.* New York: New York City Human Resources Administration, 1982.

Daiches, S. *Protective Services Risk Assessment Guide: Version II.* New York: New York City Human Resources Administration, 1983.

Flemming, A. S., Buchanan, J. G., Santos, J. F., and Rickards, L. D. *Mental Health Services for the Elderly: Report on a Survey of Community Mental Health Centers.* Vol. 1. Washington, D.C.: Action Committee to Implement the Recommendations of the 1981 White House Conference on Aging, 1984.

Hall, G. H., and Mathiasen, G. *Guide to Development of Protective Services for Older People.* Springfield, Ill.: Thomas, 1973.

Kane, R. A., and Kane, R. L. *Assessing the Elderly.* Lexington, Mass.: Lexington Books, 1981.

Katz, S., Ford, A. B., Moskowitz, R. W., Jackson, B. A., and Jaffee, M. W. "Studies of Illness in the Aged—The Index of ADL: A Standardized Measure of Biological and Psychosocial Function." *Journal of the American Medical Association,* 1963, *185,* 914–919.

Kay, D.W.K., and Bergmann, K. "Epidemiology of Mental Disorders Among the Aged in the Community." In J. E. Birren and R. B. Sloane (eds.), *Handbook of Mental Health and Aging.* Englewood Cliffs, N.J.: Prentice-Hall, 1980.

Mechanic, D. *From Advocacy to Allocation: The Evolving American Health Care System.* New York: Free Press, 1986.

Mulvey, E. P., Geller, J. L., and Roth, L. H. "The Promise and Peril of Involuntary Commitment." *American Psychologist,* 1987, *42,* 571–584.

New York City Human Resources Administration. *Short-Term Protective Orders: Implementation of a New Law.* New York: New York City Human Resources Administration, 1984.

Peters, R., Schmidt, W. C., and Miller, K. S. "Guardianship of the Elderly in Tallahassee, Florida." *The Gerontologist*, 1985, *25*, 532–538.

Regan, J. J. "Intervention Through Adult Protective Services Programs." *The Gerontologist*, 1978, *18*, 250–254.

Regan, J. J., and Springer, G. *Protective Services for the Elderly*. Washington, D.C.: U.S. Senate Special Committee on Aging, 1977.

Saunders, A. G., and Simon, M. M. "Individual Functional Assessment: An Instruction Manual." *Mental and Physical Disability Law Reporter*, 1987, *11*, 60–70.

Schmidt, W., Miller, K., Bell, W., and New, F. *Public Guardianship and the Elderly*. Cambridge, Mass.: Ballinger, 1979.

Schogt, B., and Sadavoy, J. "Assessing the Protective Service Needs of the Impaired Elderly Living in the Community." *Canadian Journal of Psychiatry*, 1987, *32*, 179–184.

Sokolovsky, J., and Cohen, C. I. "Measuring Social Interactions of the Urban Elderly: A Methodological Synthesis." *International Journal of Aging and Human Development*, 1981, *13*, 233–243.

Stephen Crystal is chair of the Division of Aging, Institute for Health, Health Care Policy, and Aging Research, and associate research professor, Rutgers University.

Edmund Dejowski is postdoctoral fellow in the Rutgers-Princeton Program in Mental Health Research at the Institute for Health, Health Care Policy, and Aging Research, Rutgers University.

A political perspective offers useful insights into the origins, organization, and impact of contemporary mental health programs. It also suggests approaches for improved advocacy, management, and delivery of services.

The Political Context of Mental Health Care

David A. Rochefort

Dorothea Dix, one of the earliest and still perhaps best-known of American mental health activists, once expressed her opinion of politicians to a friend that "they are the meanest and lowest party demagogues, shocking to say . . . the basest characters" (quoted in Brooks, 1957, p. 33). Toward the political process, she was hardly more charitable. By February 1854, the U.S. Congress had been considering Dix's proposal for the federal government to grant the states several million acres of land in support of the indigent mentally ill. (The bill eventually passed but was then vetoed by Franklin Pierce.) Dix described the legislative workings to former President Millard Fillmore as "the usual assembling and dispersion of the Senate and House, with little effected through *much speaking*—the usual amount of gossip, and the usual measure of vapid conversation and idle talk. The intrigue and selfish aims are by no means less conspicuous—with all that is so poor, so mean, so worthless" (quoted in Snyder, 1975, p. 171, emphasis in original).

Whether such judgments were overly severe can be debated (though Fillmore, for one, tended to agree); not open to argument, however, was Dix's right to state a view on the topic. Spanning a period of some four decades, her reforming activities, which resulted in the establishment or expansion of mental hospitals in twenty states, kept Dix at

D. Mechanic (ed.). *Improving Mental Health Services: What the Social Sciences Can Tell Us.*
New Directions for Mental Health Services, no. 36. San Francisco: Jossey-Bass, 1987.

the center of the political swirl, where by turns she played the roles of author of legislation, organizer, lobbyist, fund-raiser, and mobilizer of public opinion.

It seems ironic that Dix, who disdained politics and politicians, did so much to ensure that mental health programs in this country would forever after inhabit a political environment. For this nineteenth-century reformer helped spur a governmental presence, which has become greatly expanded and immeasurably more complex, in the provision and financing of mental health services that persists to the present day. The development of private health insurance notwithstanding, mental health care, particularly long-term care of the chronically mentally ill, remains largely a public expenditure. As Brown and Stockdill (1972) have commented, "This is big business. Big business means big politics, and thus, mental health must hold its place in the political arena" (p. 669). Moreover, in contrast to Dix's time, current mental health programs operate at the interface of multiple levels of government—federal, state, and local—and of public and private spheres (Morgan and Connery, 1980). Such hypertrophied relationships necessarily involve negotiation, competition, conflict, and compromise. Other complications today result from overlap in the clientele and functions of mental health versus other modern welfare state agencies (Brown and Stockdill, 1972).

Exploring these political dimensions of contemporary mental health policy making and administration is a challenging task that has attracted the attention of an eclectic, multidisciplinary group of scholars—political scientists, sociologists, historians, social workers, psychologists, and others. A review of the major concepts and research findings serves to illuminate this important subject. It also highlights certain insights and techniques relevant to improved advocacy, management, and delivery of services.

Defining a Political Perspective

A classic definition of a political perspective, as formulated by political scientist Harold Lasswell (1936), characterizes politics as the process of "who gets what, when, how." This concise dictum stresses the distribution of benefits and burdens among members of society (Isaak, 1987). David Easton (1963), who writes that politics is the "authoritative allocation of values," similarly directs attention to the distributive function but emphasizes that it takes place through the exercise of power. Also, the term "values" used in this second definition is broad enough to encompass items both tangible (goods, services, and other resources) and intangible (rights and statuses).

The political process is commonly represented as a system in which the formal institutions of government and both organized and unorganized societal groups interact in a reciprocal relationship. From society, government receives demands and support that must be translated by the mechanism of decision making into public policies. The nature and impact of these policies, in turn, determine subsequent demands and support, thus completing the circuit. The fact that different interests have conflicting goals makes difficult trade offs an inherent part of the political process, as does the sheer number of simultaneous claims made on government. And the entire system is embedded in a particular socio-economic-historical context that determines available resources and orientations to the appropriate use of public power.

The political process in society is pervasive and never ending. Although public policies can be called "the product of politics" (Shively, 1987, p. 15), there is no clear dividing line that signals where politics ends and policy begins. Indeed, politics continues as a key influence in the implementation phase of public policy making, and it can critically affect the success or failure of programs "in the field."

The Politics of Mental Health Policy Making

The functioning of the U.S. Congress as a national policy-making institution has long absorbed observers of the American political scene both before and since the time of Dorothea Dix. Central to contemporary analyses of Congress is the concept of the "subgovernment" or "iron triangle." These terms refer to the stable structure of informal relationships that commonly dictate legislative activity within specialized policy areas. Defining the points of this triangle are the committees or subcommittees assigned jurisdiction over a given substantive field, the federal administrative agency with responsibility for operating or supervising the programs up for creation or review, and affected private- or public-sector groups. The nature of involvement among these three participants tends to be symbiotic and cooperative, as each, in turn, draws from the others resources essential to its mission, whether it be technical expertise, political influence, or statutory authority. United by a common functional interest, these principals interact in a relatively closed subsystem transcending traditional institutional lines (Peters, 1986).

The Community Mental Health Centers (CMHC) Act of 1963 offers a striking illustration of the subgovernment phenomenon. A close-knit set of actors in Congress, the executive branch, state government, and the private sector collaborated to enact a sweeping reform of the public mental health system. For one, there was the National Institute of Mental Health (NIMH), which promoted the ideology of community care by means of public education programs and grants for mental health research, professional training in psychiatry and allied disciplines, and pilot community programs in the states. Supportive in this endeavor, and in the eventual review of submitted legislation, were the House and Senate Appropriations Committees, which together set NIMH's budget, and the congressional committees assigned jurisdiction for mental health policy making—the House Interstate and Foreign Commerce Committee and the Senate Committee on Labor and Welfare. Also arrayed behind the cause was a small phalanx of key interests: mental health professional associations like the American Psychiatric Association and American Psychological Association; advocacy groups such as the National Mental Health Association and National Association of State Mental Health Program Directors. Summarizing the accomplishment of this heterogeneous political alliance, Foley (1975) states that "the mental health oligopoly provided a public policy responsive to technical knowledge and congressional sentiment that it had moulded" (p. 138).

An alternative, yet in many ways complementary, perspective on this same episode of mental health policy change recognizes that institutional decision making does not occur in a historical vacuum. Rather, policy ideas often are carried to the political fore by the confluence of long-term social, intellectual, scientific, and professional currents. This is the process of "agenda access," or how an issue comes to the attention of the polity (Cobb and Elder, 1983). Working within this framework, I have examined the changing social images of the mentally ill in the post-World War II period (Rochefort, 1986). At work were a host of influences, including new awareness of the scope of the problem of mental illness, based in part on the large number of mentally disabled servicemen and veterans; mounting interest in the social aspects of the etiology and treatment of mental illnesses; exposés of the scandalous conditions within mental hospitals coupled with evidence of their debilitating effects on patients; development of powerful tranquilizing drugs that enabled new therapeutic approaches; decline of the psychiatric medical model; greater public awareness and understanding of mental illnesses; and a general "romance" with the concept of community among intellectuals and social reformers of the day. These diverse background forces were directly related to the formulation of a national community mental health policy in this period for they "converged to impart new social meaning to the plight of the mentally ill by advancing a changed image of mental illness as related to social, institutional, and biochemical factors. As mental illness lost much of its status as a psychological problem growing out of individual sources of maladjustment and deficiency, the mentally ill also increasingly came to be seen as a group that was 'deserving'—a concept of long-standing importance in social welfare policy making. This shift in perceptions led naturally to the consideration of less isolating and socially stigmatizing treatments" (Rochefort, 1986, pp. 32-33).

The politics of mental health policy making in the United States are currently in a state of flux. For example, ongoing changes in interest-group configuration and behavior may require a modification of the familiar iron triangle model of legislative operations. More descriptive, perhaps, is Heclo's (1978) notion of "issue networks" comprising an expanded number of participants acting within an atmosphere of heightened politicization. In an examination of the development of the Mental Health Systems Act of 1980 (subsequently rescinded by President Reagan), Foley and Sharfstein (1983) note the emergence since the early 1960s of new mental health constituencies having varying ideologies, aims, organization, and resources. The effect of these groups on the policy process, both in the work of the President's Commission on Mental Health and during congressional deliberations on the Mental Health Systems Act, was "a splintering of interests," "sometimes destructive competition for resources," and a "general disagreement on which recommendations to emphasize as well as on the scope of the proposed legislation" (Foley and Sharfstein, 1983, pp. 114, 122).

Growing fragmentation of interests in mental health can also be recognized in the founding in 1979 of the National Alliance for the Mentally Ill (NAMI). NAMI is a consumer organization for persons afflicted with mental illnesses and their families that has drawn clear lines between itself and clinical and administrative groups in the field. A national staff member (Hatfield, 1987) summarizes the essence of this political stance as it was adopted at the first NAMI convention: "Participants argued forcefully that other segments of the community—mental health professionals and mental health bureaucracies, in particular—had their own legitimate, but special, interests in mental health, and that these interests did not entirely coincide with those of consumers. Further, it was noted, professionals have their own power base in their professional organizations, in which nonprofessionals are not accorded membership. The NAMI was to become the lay equivalent of a professional organization for consumers" (p. 83).

Another significant development in mental health politics and policy making is the recent shift of grant-making activity under the community mental health program from the federal to the state level. With the creation of the Alcohol, Drug Abuse, and Mental Health (ADAMH) block grant in 1981, states acquired the authority, within certain general guidelines, to allocate funds and specify program priorities for local CMHC services. This relocation of decision-making responsibility to fifty subnational arenas has decided political repercussions since, as Morgan and Connery (1980) affirm, "To change the level of government at which a decision is made, or to shift the forum for decision making at a particular level, is to alter the probabilities as to what precisely will be decided. This results in large part from the simple fact that the varying institutional forms reflect and favor different political alignments" (p. 253). Moreover, the block grant program took a primary interest group under the former federally centered categorical grant system, the state mental health authorities, and gave it the ability to impose its preferences on other competing parties, notably the providers and recipients of services. Preliminary research shows a good deal of strain in the redefined state-local relationship as well as conflicting perceptions of what the evolving CMHC role should be (Logan, Rochefort, and Cook, 1985).

Mental health programs are also affected by the politics of national deficit reduction. An overriding concern with balancing the federal budget has stimulated closer scrutiny of, and constraint over, mental health expenditures. Current congressional budgeting procedures, which each year specify to committees the dollar savings needing to be realized in nonentitlement, or discretionary, programs under their jurisdiction, tend to place mental health programs in competition with other budget items, some of which may enjoy greater pressure-group and public backing (Gilbert, 1986; Bowler, 1987; Fuchs and Hoadley, 1987). Barring an unexpected rallying of congressional and executive interest in mental health issues, then, we can assume that mental health funding will increase only incrementally, if at all, in the coming years. Evidence upholding this conclusion may be found in ADAMH block grant appropriations (see Figure 1), which increased only 16 percent from fiscal years 1982 to 1987 (from $428.1 million to $495.0 million) and are still 9 percent below what the constituent programs received in fiscal year 1981 ($541.2 million) prior to consolidation (National Institute of Mental Health, 1987).

Figure 1. ADAMH Block Grant Funding, 1980–1987

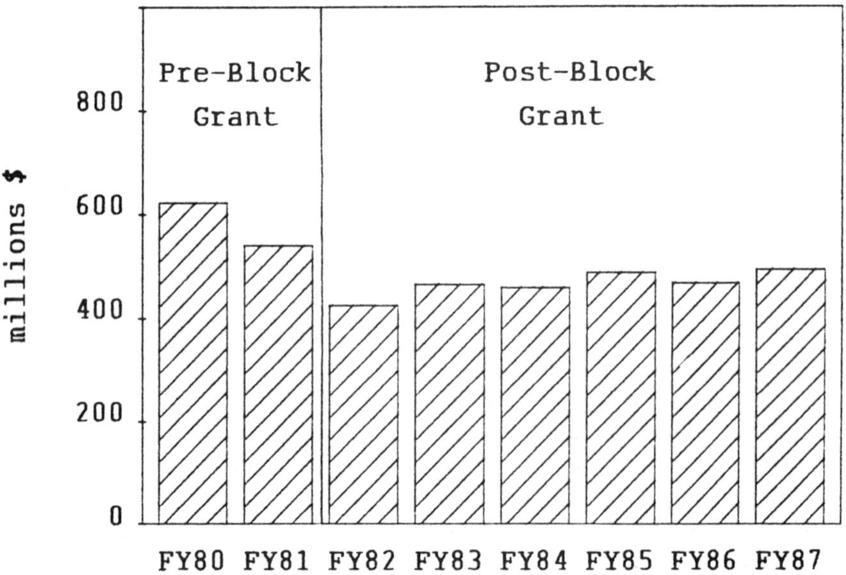

Understanding the political process through which new mental health services are established enhances the possibility of effective participation in the policy-making sphere. This discussion highlights the significance of informal as well as formal structures of governance and the different points of access, at national and state levels, that are available to mental health activists. Also, in view of today's heated competition for scarce resources, the political proponents of the mental health field should note the "balkanization" of interests in regard to mental health issues and should consider the advantages of "a more viable coalition strategy" (Ross, 1982, p. 152). For example, concerted action mobilized the mental health community in opposition to cutbacks in disability benefits for the mentally ill during the first Reagan administration, and this effort helped reverse federal policy in this area (Meyerson and Herman, 1987; Demkovich, 1984). Finally, political participants in the mental health area need to appreciate the broad social and historical forces that influence the fate of their policy proposals, as well as the characteristic waxing and waning of policy-making energies from one period to the next. Such an awareness encourages the realistic gauging of political activities for maintenance or expansion accordingly.

The Politics of Mental Health Implementation

Implementation, to paraphrase Clausewitz on war, is "the continuation of politics by other means" (Bardach, 1977, p. 85). This is the conclusion of scholars who, in recent years, have studied the process by which policy design is transformed into operating programs and services. Stimulated by disappointing results from a string of social programs over the past two decades that have jolted the liberal faith in activist government, the implementation perspective centers on the multiple social, economic, technical, bureaucratic, and organizational forces that together determine the fate of new policies. The main message of this growing body of work, according to one leading contributor (Williams, 1980), is that "the central focus of policy should be on the point of service delivery. It is not the big decisions made in the legislature or the upper reaches of executive agencies with their intrigue and glamor, but rather the management and delivery capacity of local organizations directly providing services that will determine the degree to which those served receive significant benefits" (p. ix).

Many social programs involve a crowded field of actors—public departments and agencies, private organizations, pressure groups, and providers and recipients of services. Drawing on the resources and orchestrating the behavior of this diverse, largely autonomous cast of characters require a "program assembly" process (Bardach, 1977). Often, however, different participants may try to shirk responsibility, withhold means, or redirect the program purpose. Bardach describes these political phenomena as a series of implementation games.

The game-playing framework demonstrates its appeal when applied to the implementation of the national community mental health program. One common implementation game is "Not Our Problem," in which players seek to avoid functions that are unattractive, would impose a heavy workload, or otherwise challenge their organizations. For example, many CMHCs tend to underserve severely and chronically mentally disabled clients, gravitating instead to the counseling of persons with more manageable neurotic difficulties and to delivering community consultation and education services (Dowell and Ciarlo, 1983).

The implementation game of "Resistance" refers to players' retention of elements that are critical to a program's success (Bardach, 1977). The motivation may be fundamental disagreement with the purpose of the initiative at hand or simply dissatisfaction with the terms on which a contribution is being sought. The phenomenon of community opposition to the establishment of halfway houses is a clear manifestation of social resistance to an essential service modality within the community mental health program. In this situation, the resources that are being withheld are material—the actual physical property that would be suitable as a community residence—and attitudinal—a spirit of neighborhood welcome. Researchers (Aviram and Segal, 1973; Hogan, 1986) have recorded the use of a variety of formal and informal methods to obstruct halfway house development in different locales, including petitions and public protests by neighborhood residents, restrictive zoning ordinances, and stringent application of municipal fire and building codes.

"Territory" is a well-known game of competition engaged in by players whose organizations have overlapping jurisdictions and missions. Bardach (1977) provides a choice example of the deleterious results to a community health program of unresolved issues of territory: In 1967, California enacted the Lanterman-Petris-Short Act promoting community care as an alternative to institutionalization. Formal community placement responsibilities under the act fell to the Community Services Division (CSD) of the state's Department of Social Welfare. Unfortunately, this agency stood on poor terms with the state Department of Mental Hygiene and with mental health program officials at the county level; both groups distrusted CSD and its attempts to expand patient placement activity into a broader patient advocacy mission. Given the necessity of cooperative effort among all three parties for effective patient placement, bureaucratic infighting led quickly to a deterioration in placement operations, and patients proceeded to "fall between the cracks" in service that had been opened by this dispute.

In a time of belt-tightening such as our own, effective implementation acquires greater, not lesser, importance. Williams (1980) reflects that "any new social policy directions may have to come, not from new funds, but from redirection and—more to the point—the better management of existing programs" (p. x). If anything, this statement is truer now than when it was written at the start of the decade, and nowhere more so than in the mental health policy arena.

The depiction of implementation as an intricate process of program assembly is especially pertinent for contemporary community mental health services, which intermingle a disparate group of public and private actors. Meeting the needs of the consumers of care with continuity and comprehensiveness dictates unwavering attention to issues of coordination within this sprawling nonstructure. Such administrative tools as case management, multidisciplinary treatment teams, and management information systems are part of the solution. Equally essential, however, is a steadfast commitment to mastering the administrative "countergame" and its tactics of planning, monitoring, analyzing, maneuvering, adapting, bargaining, compromising, and coercing (Bardach, 1977).

The Political Economy of Mental Health Care

As its name implies, political economy refers to the interplay between politics and economics—that is, how the institutions and transactions of each sphere impact on the other (Ferguson and Rogers, 1984; Harpham and Stone, 1982; Staniland, 1985). Of special interest for analysts on this topic is the search for a macro, holistic understanding of the welfare state that encompasses its origins, organization, funding, and effects on the social order. Within this context, mental health care is a form of public provision whose own historical development preceded, and then was transformed by, modern federal interventionism.

Mental health has proved rich terrain for the application and further refinement of basic political-economic tenets regarding the "interconnectedness" of social welfare activities across a spectrum of nominally distinct policy areas. According to this perspective, deinstitutionalization cannot be understood apart from the stimulus of income-maintenance programs, like Supplemental Security Income and Social Security Disability Insurance, which provided a means of financially supporting the mentally ill in the community and permitted a shifting of costs from state to federal levels (Scull, 1976, 1977; Lerman, 1985; Rose, 1979). In the same way, federally matched Medicaid funding made it virtually irresistible, from an economic point of view, for states to transfer thousands of mental patients from public hospitals to nursing homes. The strength of the economic incentives posed by such programs is evident in empirical analyses of deinstitutionalization patterns. One careful comparative study, for example, found hospital inpatient declines at the state level to correlate much more strongly with Medicaid payments than with measures of CMHC service activity (Gronfein, 1985).

Prominent within the field of political economy is a Marxist view of the state as an instrument for advancing class interests (Staniland, 1985). When applied to the mental health system, this approach interprets deinstitutionalization as a policy aimed at social control of a deviant population at minimal cost and subsidization of a new social-medical-industrial complex of nursing homes, drug manufacturers, board-and-care facilities, and other proprietary enterprises. Scull (1976), for example, observes that "an effort is under way to transform 'social junk' into a commodity from which various 'professionals' and entrepreneurs can extract a profit" (p. 209). Aside from its obviously cynical quality, such a depiction seems to attribute an unrealistic coherency to the disjointed American social policy apparatus. Emphasizing the spasmodic, unplanned character of a social reform movement like deinstitutionalization, others relate the flow of dollars and clients in contemporary mental health to inadvertence and to the ungoverned complexity of the social service system, whose cross-level, cross-program interactions produce unforeseen, sometimes undesired, consequences (Gronfein, 1985; Lerman, 1985; Mechanic, 1985).

Important implications for program development follow from this political-economy analysis. The centralized control and unity of purpose lacking in public mental health policy at the national level must somehow be supplied elsewhere in the system if the chronically mentally ill are to be adequately supported in the community setting. The most innovative responses to this problem have involved the creation of substate management structures having superintendency over a unified budget for meeting the comprehensive service needs—mental health and social—of a defined group of enrollees or geographic population (Mechanic, 1985). Examples include Integrated Mental Health, Inc., of New York's Monroe and Livingston counties, Arizona's Regional Authorities, Wisconsin's Dane County system, and the Program for the Chronically Mentally Ill jointly sponsored by the Robert Wood Johnson Foundation and U.S. Department of Housing and Urban Development (Dickey and Goldman, 1986; Mechanic, 1986). Continued experimentation and evaluation will be necessary to assess the performance of these and alternate program models with respect to different types of clients, different service modalities, overall cost effectiveness, and "transportability" to other settings.

Conclusion

Politics has been called the most popular of all spectator sports. For those in the mental health field, however, watching from the stands while the game is being played would be a regrettable indulgence, for it is the political process in society that determines what resources will be allocated to mental health services and, in large measure, how these services will be organized and whether they will achieve their intended effects. Though it may be, as Dorothea Dix had occasion to observe, that participation in the political arena is not always a gratifying experience, there can be no other option for effective advocacy within our democratic system—and this, her lengthy public career tells us, Dix also knew. Murray Levine, author of *The History and Politics of Community Mental Health* (1981), succinctly makes the point when stating that "politics is not wrong or bad. It is inevitable. It is bad or wrong only if we blind ourselves to those inevitabilities" (p. 9).

References

Aviram, U., and Segal, S. "Exclusion of the Mentally Ill: Reflection on an Old Problem in a New Context." *Archives of General Psychiatry*, 1973, *29*, 126–131.

Bardach, E. *The Implementation Game: What Happens After a Bill Becomes a Law.* Cambridge, Mass.: M.I.T. Press, 1977.

Bowler, M. K. "Changing Politics of Federal Health Insurance Programs." *PS*, 1987, *20*, 202–211.

Brooks, G. *Three Wise Virgins.* New York: Dutton, 1957.

Brown, B. M., and Stockdill, J. W. "The Politics of Mental Health." In S. E. Golann and C. Eisdorfer (eds.), *Handbook of Community Mental Health.* New York: Appleton-Century-Crofts, 1972.

Cobb, R. W., and Elder, C. D. *Participation in American Politics: The Dynamics of Agenda-Building.* (2nd ed.) Baltimore, Md.: Johns Hopkins University Press, 1983.

Demkovich, L. E. "Administration About-Face on Disability Could Be a Political Blessing in Disguise." *National Journal*, April 28, 1984, pp. 823–825.

Dickey, B., and Goldman, H. H. "Public Health Care for the Chronically Mentally Ill: Financing Operating Costs: Issues and Options for Local Leadership." *Administration in Mental Health*, 1986, *14*, 63–77.

Dowell, D. A., and Ciarlo, J. A. "Overview of the Community Mental Health Centers Program from an Evaluation Perspective." *Community Mental Health Journal*, 1983, *19*, 95–125.

Easton, D. *The Political System.* New York: Knopf, 1963.

Ferguson, T., and Rogers, J. "Introduction." In T. Ferguson, and J. Rogers (eds.), *The Political Economy: Readings in the Politics and Economics of American Public Policy.* Armonk, N.Y.: Sharpe, 1984.

Foley, H. A. *Community Mental Health Legislation: The Formative Process.* Lexington, Mass.: Heath, 1975.

Foley, H. A., an Sharfstein, S. S. *Madness and Government: Who Care for the Mentally Ill?* Washington, D.C.: American Psychiatric Press, 1983.

Fuchs, B. C., and Hoadley, J. F. "Reflections from Inside the Beltway: How Congress and the President Grapple with Health Policy." *PS*, 1987, *20*, 212–220.

Gilbert, R. C. "Gramm-Rudman: What It Means to Mental Health and Domestic Spending." *Administration in Mental Health*, 1986, *13*, 249–259.

Gronfein, W. "Incentives and Intentions in Mental Health Policy: A Comparison of the Medicaid and Community Mental Health Programs." *Journal of Health and Social Behavior*, 1985, *26*, 192–206.

Harpham, E. J., and Stone, A. "Volume Editors' Introduction: The Study of Political Economy." In A. Stone, and E. J. Harpham (eds.), *Political Economy of Public Policy.* Newbury Park, Calif.: Sage, 1982.

Hatfield, A. B. "The National Journal of Mental Health, 1987, *15*, 79-93.

Heclo, H. "Issue Networks and the Executive Establishment." In A. King (ed.), *The New American Political System*. Washington, D.C.: American Enterprise Institute, 1978.

Hogan, R. "Community Opposition to Group Homes." *Social Science Quarterly*, 1986, *67*, 442-449.

Isaak, A. *An Introduction to Politics*. Glenview, Ill: Scott, Foresman, 1987.

Lasswell, H. D. *Politics: Who Gets What, When, How*. New York: McGraw-Hill, 1936.

Lerman, P. "Deinstitutionalization and Welfare Policies." *Annals of the American Academy of Political and Social Science*, 1985, *479*, 132-155.

Levine, M. *The History and Politics of Community Mental Health*. New York: Oxford University Press, 1981.

Logan, B. M., Rochefort, D. A., and Cook, E. W. "Block Grants for Mental Health: Elements of the State Response." *Journal of Public Health Policy*, 1985, *6*, 476-492.

Mechanic, D. "Mental Health and Social Policy: Initiatives for the 1980s." *Health Affairs*, 1985, *4*, 75-88.

Mechanic, D. "The Challenge of Chronic Mental Illness: A Retrospective and Prospective View." *Hospital and Community Psychiatry*, 1986, *37*, 891-896.

Meyerson, A. T., and Herman, G. H. "Systems Resistance to the Chronic Patient." In A. T. Meyerson (ed.), *Barriers to Treating the Chronic Mentally Ill*. New Directions for Mental Health Services, no. 33. San Francisco: Jossey-Bass, 1987.

Morgan, J. A., Jr., and Connery, R. H. "The Governmental System." In S. Feldman (ed.), *The Administration of Mental Health Services*. (2nd ed.) Springfield, Ill.: Thomas, 1980.

National Institute of Mental Health. Data provided by the Division of Education and Service Systems Liaison, State Planning and Resource Development Branch, Rockville, Md., 1987.

Peters, B. G. *American Public Policy: Promise and Performance*. (2nd ed.) Chatham, N.J.: Chatham House, 1986.

Rochefort, D. A. *American Social Welfare Policy: Dynamics of Formulation and Change*. Boulder, Colo.: Westview Press, 1986.

Rose, S. M. "Deciphering Deinstitutionalization: Complexities in Policy and Program Analysis." *Milbank Memorial Fund Quarterly*, 1979, *57*, 218-249.

Ross, E. C. "Development of Constituencies and Their Organizations: Public Policy Formulation at the National Level." In J. J. Bevilacqua (ed.), *Changing Government Policies for the Mentally Disabled*. Cambridge, Mass.: Ballinger, 1982.

Scull, A. T. "The Decarceration of the Mentally Ill: A Critical View." *Politics and Society*, 1976, *6*, 173-211.

Scull, A. T. *Decarceration: Community Treatment and the Deviant—A Radical View*. Englewood Cliffs, N.J.: Prentice-Hall, 1977.

Shively, W. P. *Power and Choice: An Introduction to Political Science*. New York: Random House, 1987.

Snyder, C. M. *The Lady and the President: The Letters of Dorothea Dix and Millard Fillmore*. Lexington: University Press of Kentucky, 1975.

Staniland, M. *What Is Political Economy? A Study of Social Theory and Underdevelopment*. New Haven, Conn.: Yale University Press, 1985.

Williams, W. *The Implementation Perspective: A Guide for Managing Social Service Delivery Programs*. Berkeley: University of California Press, 1980.

David A. Rochefort is a former postdoctoral fellow in the Rutgers-Princeton Program in Mental Health Research at the Institute for Health, Health Care Policy, and Aging Research, Rutgers University, and is presently a member of the political science department at Northeastern University.

Because the structure of financing options for the care of the seriously mentally ill affects the patterns of care received, mental health care reform must begin with changes to the financing structures.

Financing Care for the Seriously Mentally Ill

Jeffrey Rubin

Increasingly, efforts to reform the mental health care system begin with changes in the way mental health services are financed. When financing structures are established, several fundamental decisions must be made, including determining the program eligibility criteria, the benefits provided by each program, and the amount paid for specific services, as well as identifying the providers and defining the way they will be reimbursed. These decisions affect the kinds and amounts of mental health care received and who receives such care.

In this chapter, I offer a brief overview of available mechanisms for financing services for the seriously mentally ill. Then I describe some of the recent proposals to reform the financing and organization of mental health care. The potential pitfalls and inadequacies in these plans will be noted, and suggestions for changes will be made.

The Current Picture

Currently there is a vast array of funding sources to pay for care and services for the seriously mentally ill. These sources can be categorized any number of ways, and one important distinction is between private and public programs.

D. Mechanic (ed.). *Improving Mental Health Services: What the Social Sciences Can Tell Us.*
New Directions for Mental Health Services, no. 36. San Francisco: Jossey-Bass, 1987.

Private sources include individual earnings, family income, and privately purchased health and disability insurance. Public sources can be subdivided into federal, state, and local. The funds can be made available in many forms; for example, there are cash payments that an individual is free to allocate however he or she wishes. Other programs can restrict the use of funds to pay for certain services. Alternatively, programs can be designed to pay providers directly for services supplied to eligible persons, or public entities may hire the employees and deliver the care themselves.

The rules and regulations governing these programs are fairly complex and have been discussed by others on numerous occasions (Parry, 1985; Burt and Pittman, 1985). Only a brief review of the major programs is offered here as the basis for examining several proposals for reform.

State Programs. The most obvious source of funding for mental health care is direct state allocations to build, maintain, and operate hospitals for the mentally ill. Though the relative importance of these facilities has declined, they still represent a visible and costly form of care. Most reform options focus on ways to shift funding away from inpatient care toward community-based programs.

Data from the National Institute of Mental Health (NIMH) indicate that in January 1984 there were 277 state and county mental hospitals as compared to a total of 323 ten years earlier—a decline of 14.2 percent (Greene and others, 1986). The change in the number of inpatient beds over the same period was even more substantial, declining nearly 54 percent to a total of 128,626 in January 1984. Yet total expenditures in these hospitals reached nearly $5.5 billion in 1983, resulting in maintenance expenditures per inpatient of $127.04 per day or $46,370 per year. In constant dollars, costs have increased over 3.5 times, from $9.87 to $35.56 per day in the past fifteen years.

The extent to which state and county hospitals are utilized, especially for short-term hospitalization, varies considerably across the states. Beyond the need for a protective environment for the dangerous or gravely disabled mentally ill, there are economic and legal reasons for both the continued reliance on and the rising costs of public mental hospitals. Often, these facilities are a major source of economic support for their localities; the economic impact of closing a facility or reducing employment is often cited as a justification for keeping a hospital open. It is also true that, while a policy of deinstitutionalization has lowered the average daily census, the remaining population in state institutions is, on the average, more severely impaired than was once the case; the rising real costs of care may reflect the need to provide more services per patient. Furthermore, legal decisions have established levels of adequate care that must be met for persons involuntarily institutionalized, thereby further increasing the cost of care (Weiner, 1985).

States affect the financing of community programs, as well, through direct allocations and through the use of federal funds passed to states as part of a block grant. These direct allocations to providers, or, in some cases, to county agencies to allocate to providers, form the basic structure of a community-based system of care.

The mechanisms for distributing these funds vary across states. In some cases, funds are allocated to community mental health centers in return for specific services in a kind of contract arrangement. In other cases, per-capita allocations are made to counties based on estimated rates of mental illness. In other instances, performance-based allocations are made.

Federal Programs. At the federal level, three mechanisms are used to provide financial support to the seriously mentally ill. One mechanism, block grant allocations to states, has already been noted. Other programs provide direct cash payments to individuals; these programs include Social Security Disability Insurance (SSDI), Supplemental Security Insurance (SSI), the Veterans Administration (VA), and welfare programs.

A third category of programs uses federal funds to finance services individuals need. Medicaid and Medicare are the primary examples. Like the welfare programs, Medicaid is partly a state-supported program and partly a federal-supported program. Under Medicaid, states have many options in regard to eligibility criteria and covered benefits, which results in different treatment for the seriously mentally ill simply on the basis of where they reside. On the other hand, Medicare has a single set of rules governing all participants; the same eligibility and benefit criteria apply in all states.

These programs differ in some other significant respects, as well. For example, Medicare is considered a social insurance program with eligibility based on prior contributions. Medicaid is a welfare program where eligibility depends on meeting certain income and disability tests. Medicare primarily finances health care services for persons over age sixty-five. Two other groups are eligible for Medicare coverage: recipients of SSDI for two years and persons with end-stage renal disease. Thus, many of the young chronically mentally ill who can become eligible for SSDI through their own contributions while working or as dependents of persons eligible for Social Security benefits may also be eligible for Medicare (Lubitz and Pine, 1986).

Both Medicare and Medicaid were patterned after the private health insurance programs in force in the midsixties. Reimbursement operated on a cost-based system in which providers were paid on a fee-for-service basis. This financing mechanism was largely responsible for an explosion in costs far beyond what was envisioned. Another consequence was a reliance on hospital-based care.

Thus, neither Medicare nor Medicaid was especially suited to meeting the needs of the seriously mentally ill. For example, many of the mentally ill may be capable of returning to work for short periods of time, in which case their earnings may lead to disqualification from SSDI or SSI benefits and consequently from Medicare and Medicaid as well. Also, treatment of a serious mental illness may require less reliance on medical types of services (such as inpatient care) and more support from social, rehabilitation, and supervisory services.

Many believe that one example of how financial incentives in public programs can yield the wrong kind of service is Medicaid's coverage of nursing home care (Gronfein, 1985). Unlike Medicare, Medicaid will cover lengthy stays in nursing homes. When a lack of community services, combined with a lack of available housing, forces someone eligible for Medicaid to turn elsewhere, the nursing home often becomes a refuge. But nursing homes often are not equipped to treat serious mental illness, in part because reimbursement rules limit specialization in mental health care. Many professionals regard this sort of "transinstitutionalization" as inappropriate and potentially harmful; others argue that nursing homes could become a more constructive element in a mental health care system (Shadish and Bootzin, 1981).

The nursing home portion of the Medicaid program was created primarily to meet the needs of many poor families whose older members were becoming frail and unable to live in the community. The program was not designed to meet the needs of the mentally ill. Yet, when deinstitutionalization rushed to the community persons who had been hospitalized or others who would have been hospitalized under previous commitment criteria, the lack of community resources forced families and medical and social service workers to seek alternative sources. Medicaid proved a convenient source for funding care, even if the locus of treatment had to be the nursing home.

As for other categories of federal support, one estimate suggests that states spent $231 million of the Alcohol, Drug Abuse, and Mental Health block grant in 1984 for the mentally ill (Burt and Pittman, 1985). In real dollar terms, this figure represents a substantial reduction from comparable programs just five years earlier.

Veterans Administration programs, funds from the federal-state vocational rehabilitation program, and a wide array of federally supported housing programs for persons with low incomes also offer some financial support for the mentally ill. However, eligibility requirements vary in each program, contributing to the confusion surrounding the extent and adequacy of resources available to the seriously mentally ill. In fact, there are no cross-sectional or longitudinal studies of exactly how much and which types of federal, state, and local support this population receives. Such research could determine what gaps exist for which persons. To date, most of the criticism of the quasi system that exists to finance care and services for the seriously mentally ill stems either from aggregate observations about such matters as the extent of nursing home use and the coverage of the mentally ill in SSDI and SSI or from anecdotal evidence about the inability of providers to obtain funding for certain services.

Because payments for services for the seriously mentally ill are often lumped together with other mental health or disability expenditure data, it is difficult to obtain an accurate estimate of the public cost of serious mental illness. One of the few available estimates puts the total figure in 1983 at $11.1 billion with 59.5 percent coming from the federal government, 37.8 percent from state sources, and the remaining 2.7 percent from local governments (Dickey and Goldman, 1986).

Private Sources. Talbott and Sharfstein (1986) suggest that between 49 percent and 65 percent of the 1.7 to 2.4 million chronically mentally ill live with their families. Those who are dependents of employed persons are likely to be covered for certain mental health services through the employee's health insurance coverage. Often this coverage is limited; for example, there may be limits on the total lifetime costs that an insurer will pay for treatment of a mental health problem. In other cases, the deductibles and coinsurance for mental health services are higher than those applied to other health care services. Also, restrictions may be imposed on the type of provider who will be reimbursed.

In cases where a child is totally disabled, some insurance plans cover dependent children beyond the age at which benefits would normally terminate, but some policies have restricted this extension of coverage to exclude those who are disabled due to a mental illness (Rubin, forthcoming). In these situations, a family will either have to spend large sums of money to finance care, have the child institutionalized, or attempt to have the child qualify for welfare assistance and Medicaid benefits.

Even when insurance coverage is available for the mentally ill, policies may alter the relative prices of different forms of care and hence distort the pattern of choices people would make if all services were treated the same. These relative price differences tend to bias care toward institutional-based services and away from community-based care. Another consequence of private insurance design is that the mentally ill are encouraged to seek more medically oriented forms of care and less social service assistance than is appropriate. Again, these problems stem from the effort to adapt the basic health insurance model to a set of mental conditions that, in their effects on the individual, are very different from physical illness.

Private health insurance is in the midst of major reforms designed to redirect much health care to less costly outpatient systems. Health maintenance organizations (HMOs) with capitated payments, prospective payment with reimbursement for hospital stays based on diagnosis, and preferred provider arrangements are some of the current strategies being implemented. In part, these mechanisms are designed to induce providers to produce care more efficiently and to encourage patients to obtain care in less costly settings. For the most part, however, the seriously mentally ill will not be affected by these reforms: first, because a large portion of expenditures for this group comes from public cash assistance programs; second, because a significant portion of funding comes from publicly produced services, such as state hospitals and VA facilities, which are largely exempt from these reforms; and third, because some of the prospective systems have excluded psychiatric care from their reimbursement system.

Options for Reform

This section presents some of the most significant financing reforms now being proposed and tried.

Pooling Existing Funds. One of the most extensive reforms was recently outlined in an article by Talbott and Sharfstein (1986). One of their goals is the creation of a comprehensive system of care for the seriously mentally ill that would fund the range of services provided by a full-care institution. Another requirement is the need to fix responsibility for care. Talbott and Sharfstein also seek systemic changes that would direct patients to community care while giving patients a choice in selection of providers. Another goal for the system is to give providers incentives to be cost effective and to produce high-quality services.

The authors' plan includes the creation of a new federal entitlement program funded by pooling the existing funds currently spent on behalf of the chronically mentally ill. These funds would be channeled to local programs on a capitation basis; in other words, using population, incidence, prevalence, and cost data, a dollar amount for each funding district would be determined. Each state's initial grant would be no smaller than its current share of funds from existing programs. States would be required to set up a coordinating agency to allocate the funds and to develop a system of care. A key element is that the relative prices for community and institutional care would not be biased by the plan. Whichever care the managing agency decided to provide would be based on its true cost, the patient's needs, and the relative quality of care.

Critics of the plan (Rubenstein, Koyanagi, and Manes, 1987) point out that one of the dilemmas posed by establishing a new entitlement program is the separation of the mentally ill from other disadvantaged groups in the political struggle for funds. They argue that, when this separation has occurred in the past, the mentally ill have never been very successful. In addition, by pooling cash payments, the plan will deprive the mentally ill of the dignity and positive reinforcement that goes with making spending decisions. Then, too, these funds are used by the seriously mentally ill to purchase necessities; the proposal would put local managers in the position of having to allocate funds to the mentally ill for food, clothing, shelter, and other personal needs.

As an alternative, Rubenstein, Koyanagi, and Manes suggest reforming the existing poorly designed spending programs, and they point to past changes that have improved SSDI and SSI and broadened Medicaid to include financing for case management and community programs.

In reply, Sharfstein and Talbott (1987) cite current inadequacies in funding mental health care and a need to create, in the community, some semblance of the managed system of care associated with institutions. The former point is perhaps most telling. By claiming that insufficient funds have been available, the authors seem to be suggesting that their proposal requires an injection of new funds. This carries them beyond the notion of pooling existing resources, and it highlights a distinction critical to any discussion of financing reforms: Changing the way existing dollars are spent is a different approach than changing the numbers of people who are eligible for these funds or the amounts they are eligible to receive.

The Monroe and Livingston County Plan. A variation of the pooling concept has been developed for testing within two counties in New York (Lehman, 1987). The agency to be used in this experiment is similar to the kind of local organization envisioned in the Talbott and Sharfstein proposal. A nonprofit corporation will be created, will receive a capitation payment, and will have responsibility for coordinating care. Three types of patients, each with different needs, have been identified, and varying amounts of money will be allocated to the agency for each type. Corresponding to each patient type is a set of required services that the agency must purchase. Community mental health centers in the two counties will act as lead agencies to provide and pay for the care of persons under the capitation system.

Lehman (1987) notes that one problem with this system is the difficulty of defining the risk groups and establishing capitation rates. The cost for meeting patients' varying needs will differ, but too many rate variations might inspire participants to categorize people only into the highest possible capitation group. There also needs to be a mechanism by which people move in and out of this kind of system. In a typical HMO, the individual is free to exit and enter the program and, in effect, take his or her capitation payment along. In this experiment, the lead agency appears to be responsible for deciding when someone will be eligible for the program and when the eligibility, and presumably the capitation payment, will cease.

Mental Health Authority. Another alternative to providing care and treatment for the severely mentally ill is being developed by the Robert Wood Johnson Foundation and the U.S. Department of Housing and Urban Development (Aiken, Somers, and Shore, 1986). Currently being initiated in nine large cities, the basic goal is to establish a single mental health authority to supervise and manage the care of the seriously mentally ill. These authorities would be organized to bear the administrative, fiscal, and service responsibility necessary to coordinate and integrate mental health and other needed services. As with the other programs, this plan is based on the perception that the wide range of available funding sources makes the current system unmanageable for the mentally ill and their advocates.

Other Options and Some Doubts. There are a great many variations on the basic themes of coordinating care, providing incentives for community care, and meeting the whole spectrum of social as well as medical needs of the seriously mentally ill. One version would utilize an HMO model and create private organizations to receive a capitation payment for each person they agree to accept and for which they will provide a specified range of services. Other variations are described in a recent survey of such programs by Dickey and Goldman (1986).

Beyond the political and design problems of pooled and managed systems of care, a new dilemma has been raised concerning the effectiveness of case management. A report of an experimental case management system in Texas calls into question some of the premises behind this approach (Franklin and others, 1987).

In the Texas project, a group of chronically mentally ill persons were randomly assigned to an experimental group and a control group. Those in the experimental group received case management services, while the control group had to locate mental health services through existing mechanisms. To evaluate the effectiveness of case management, the researchers assessed the clients twelve months later with respect to service utilization, cost of care, and quality of life.

The authors acknowledge some difficulties in tracking all clients and the potential for incorrect conclusions based on the brief period during which the program operated. Though the results must be interpreted cautiously, the study produced some interesting data. Those clients receiving case management averaged more than twice as many community-based services as those in the control group. The groups differed little in terms of medication, but the experimental group used substantially more social-economic services, short-term therapy services, and services under the category labeled "other," which included treatment planning, case consultation, referrals and screening services.

The authors found little difference between the groups in their satisfaction with their homes. On several objective measures, both groups experienced only minor changes. The experimental group, however, experienced a 7 percent decline in the number who were unemployed, while the control group had a 10 percent increase in the number who were unemployed. Both groups improved on their quality of life measures over the course of the project, with the experimental group doing slightly better.

The higher cost of serving the experimental group and the lack of substantial improvements in quality of life measures raise doubts about the appropriateness, at this time, of implementing major reforms that include a critical role for case management.

Conclusion

How society chooses to finance and organize care of the seriously mentally ill will determine how many and what kinds of services they receive. Choosing a financing system is not a task to be completed after a program has been designed. As mental health professionals have come to realize the ways in which financing influences the allocation and distribution of services, they have begun to propose changes in the existing financing structure. Some proposals involve incremental changes to programs already in place. Other options involve reapportioning available funds in a dramatic fashion. Sometimes proponents of specific plans are seeking more funds, either to serve more people or to provide more services for those already eligible for support. Regardless of the direction taken, an understanding of how all participants can be expected to respond to new financing arrangements is critical to creating a proposal that can effectively achieve the goals of its proponents.

References

Aiken, L. H., Somers, S., and Shore, M. F. "Private Foundations in Health Affairs: A Case Study of the Development of a National Initiative for the Chronically Mentally Ill." *American Psychologist*, 1986, *41*, 1290-1295.

Burt, M. R., and Pittman, K. J. *Testing the Social Safety Net*. Washington, D.C.: Urban Institute Press, 1985.

Dickey, B., and Goldman, H. H. "Public Health Care for the Chronically Mentally Ill: Financing Operating Costs." *Administration in Mental Health*, 1986, *14* (2), 63-77.

Franklin, J. L., Solovitz, B., Mason, M., Clemons, J. R., and Miller, G. E. "An Evaluation of Case Management." *American Journal of Public Health*, 1987, 77 (6), 674-678.

Greene, S., Witkin, M. J., Atay, J., Fell, A., and Manderscheid, R. W. *State and County Mental Hospitals, United States, 1982-83 and 1983-84, with Trend Analyses from 1973-74 to 1983-84*. Mental Health Statistical Note no. 176. Rockville, Md.: National Institute of Mental Health, 1986.

Gronfein, W. "Incentives and Intentions in Mental Health Policy: A Comparison of the Medicaid and Community Mental Health Programs." *Journal of Health and Social Behavior*, 1985, *26*, 192-206.

Lehman, A. F. "Capitation Payment and Mental Health Care: A Review of the Opportunities and Risks." *Hospital and Community Psychiatry*, 1987, *38* (1), 31-38.

Lubitz, J., and Pine, P. "Health Care Use by Medicare's Disabled Enrollees." *Health Care Financing Review*, 1986, 7 (4), 19-31.

Parry, J. "Rights and Entitlements in the Community." In S. J. Brakel, J. Parry, and B. A. Weiner (eds.), *The Mentally Disabled and the Law*. (3rd ed.) Chicago: American Bar Foundation, 1985.

Rubenstein, L. S., Koyanagi, C., and Manes, J. "Mental Health Funding." *Hospital and Community Psychiatry*, 1987, *38* (4), 410-411.

Rubin, J. "Discrimination and Insurance Coverage of the Mentally Ill." In R. Scheffler and T. McGuire (eds.), *Advances in Health Economics and Health Services Research*. Vol. 8. Greenwich, Conn.: JAI Press, forthcoming.

Shadish, W. R., and Bootzin, R. R. "Nursing Homes and Chronic Mental Patients." *Schizophrenia Bulletin*, 1981, 7 (3), 488-498.

Sharfstein, S. S., and Talbott, J. A. "In Reply." *Hospital and Community Psychiatry*, 1987, *38* (4), 411.

Talbott, J. A., and Sharfstein, S. S. "A Proposal for Future Funding of Chronic and Episodic Mental Illness." *Hospital and Community Psychiatry*, 1986, *37* (11), 1126-1130.

Weiner, B. A. "Treatment Rights." In S. J. Brakel, J. Parry, and B. A. Weiner (eds.), *The Mentally Disabled and the Law*. (3rd ed.) Chicago: American Bar Foundation, 1985.

Jeffrey Rubin is associate professor of economics and is a member of the Institute for Health, Health Care Policy, and Aging Research, Rutgers University.

*Outpatient commitment has recently developed as a legal
device for maintaining noncompliant chronically mentally
ill patients in the community and for preventing the revolving-
door syndrome, but this new approach presents difficult
problems in reconciling the liberty of patients with
their treatment needs.*

Outpatient Commitment for the Chronically Mentally Ill: Law and Policy

Alexander D. Brooks

The past two decades have seen major legal reforms in the mental health system, most of them directed at improving care and reducing compulsory hospitalization. In cases of involuntary civil commitment, more restrictive standards, such as an emphasis on dangerousness as a requirement and protective procedures that require hearings, the right to a lawyer, and other due-process guarantees have contributed substantially to a reduction in long-term hospitalizations. Such novel legal concepts as the right to treatment and the right to refuse treatment now protect hospitalized patients against previously common abuse and neglect. One of the consequences of these legal changes has been the deinstitutionalization of thousands of mental patients throughout the country (Brooks, 1979), which in turn has presented many new legal and social problems.

Deinstitutionalization has always been a major objective of legal reform. Lawyers, in acting against hospitalization, have hoped that the large-scale discharge of mental patients from hospitals would inevitably generate appropriate responses in the community for their care. Lawyers and mental health professionals alike anticipated that communities would provide acceptable housing, treatment, employment opportunities,

D. Mechanic (ed.). *Improving Mental Health Services: What the Social Sciences Can Tell Us.*
New Directions for Mental Health Services, no. 36. San Francisco: Jossey-Bass, 1987.

crisis intervention, case management, and other services that would make community living for the chronically mentally ill feasible.

These hopes, as we all know, have been disappointed so far: Adequate support has not been forthcoming. As a result, a large proportion of discharged mental patients have been effectively abandoned (Lamb, 1984).

A variety of solutions for this sorry state of affairs has been presented. One, favored primarily by psychiatrists but disfavored by libertarians, is the rehospitalization of those mentally ill persons who are unable to "survive in the community." This approach has taken the form of statutory amendments that significantly enlarge the category of persons subject to involuntary civil commitment, thus making it feasible to commit previously uncommittable nondangerous mentally ill persons whose mental health and survival capacities are in the process of deteriorating. A few states, notably Washington, have experimented with this approach, which Treffert (1985) has labeled the "fourth standard." The reinstitutionalization solution has been criticized as both inhumane and unfeasible. A recent study of the Washington state experience by Durham and LaFond (1985) indicates that implementation of the so-called fourth standard there has resulted in a substantial increase in civil involuntary commitment accompanied by extensive hospital overcrowding and a decline in the quality of hospital care and treatment.

A second proposed approach is to place no constraints or conditions on the chronically mentally ill in the community but to increase and improve services for them. This position reflects the widely held view that community living for the chronically mentally ill has not failed because of inherent unworkability but rather because it has not been adequately implemented. The argument is made that homelessness, bag ladies, incidents of violence, and mentally ill persons roaming the streets and sleeping in doorways are the inevitable result of lack of services. If sufficient services and housing were provided, most of the problems now posed by deinstitutionalization, including noncompliance with medications, would be resolved (Schwartz and Costanzo, 1987). Toward this end, some states, local communities, and private foundations have taken the initiative to provide such services. Lawyers have attempted, with modest success, to establish a legal right, based mainly on a liberal interpretation of preexisting statutes, to care and treatment in the community for the chronically mentally ill. In some communities, litigation has actually resulted in more substantial funding. And there is indeed strong evidence that the provision of appropriate services substantially stabilizes many of the chronically mentally ill (Mechanic, 1986).

The third approach—and the focus of this chapter—is outpatient commitment. This approach is based on the view that, within the larger group of chronically mentally ill persons in the community, there is a subset of persons in need of more constraint and structure than the community typically can provide. Most of these are the so-called revolving-door patients, who go in and out of mental hospitals with excessive frequency. While in the community, these patients become destabilized and dangerous to themselves or others. They are then hospitalized and treated with antipsychotic medications. As they are restored to functionality, they become eligible for discharge. If no longer dangerous to themselves or others, their continued confinement becomes illegal and their continued hospitalization no longer appropriate. Moreover, their beds are needed for more acute cases and for those patients who cannot be stabilized.

In the past, most stabilized patients have been discharged without any conditions placed on them. Many of them, relieved of any compulsion to take their crucial medications, stop doing so. Community support, including outreach services, that might help them to continue the medications, are inadequate or nonexistent. The patients decompensate, again become dangerous, and are finally rehospitalized, in some cases after committing acts of violence that outrage the community. For many chronically mentally ill persons, this has become a vicious cycle. Everyone suffers, particularly the mentally ill person, who may lose a job and friends and suffer from a sense of failure. Others who suffer are his or her family and friends, potential victims of violence, and society at large.

Evidence suggests that, even if there were an appropriate availability of mental health services in the community, there would still be a substantial number of chronic patients who would be noncompliant with treatment, most particularly with medications. For that reason, improving services, while essential, is not a complete answer. Some form of pressure, as minimal as possible, seems necessary to ensure compliance.

Patterns of Noncompliance

A brief analysis of noncompliance may be useful at this point. While there is no such thing as a stereotypical noncomplier, noncompliant patients, for our purposes, may be divided roughly into three groups. The first consists of those who would comply if encouraged but for whom positive reinforcements are lacking. For these patients, medications may be too expensive, the mental health center inaccessible, and friends or family unavailable to act as reminders. If adequate outreach, transportation, funds, and family encouragement were provided, compliance would tend to follow. Such patients, many of whom are "minimally disturbed," need very little pressure. Outpatient commitment may be a relatively benevolent way to supply what these patients need and are willing to accept.

A second group of noncompliers are those who, once restored, regard themselves as no longer in need of medication and, despite admonitions, neglect to take it, as a result of which they decompensate. Ironically, most of these patients promise to take their medications at the time they are discharged from the hospital and seem to have every intention of doing so. But the motive to comply and the insight, neither of which is very high in the first place, diminish when the structure of the hospital is removed and these patients become subject to the stresses of community living. Their subsequent noncompliance is usually a consequence of irrational misperceptions resulting from their mental illness, a condition that antipsychotic medications often fail to address as dramatically as they do delusions and hallucinations (Davis, 1985). Many think they are not really mentally ill or that the medications are unnecessary. These patients require some coercion if they are not to backslide. Indeed, it has been argued that some of these patients, when pressured into accepting their medications, become symptom-free for long periods of time and grateful for relief from mental illness (Geller, 1986). For such patients, outpatient commitment seems essential.

A third group consists of patients who do appreciate the benefit of medications but who suffer severely from dysphoric and other distressing side effects. Eventually they refuse to take their medications. The noncompliance of such patients is not irrational in the sense that the patients lack insight. They are torn between their recognition of the value of medications and an understandable unwillingness to tolerate the physical anguish that medications impose on them. Many of these patients may appropriately see that, for them, the benefit is offset by the risks. Many of these patients seesaw back and forth, taking their medications at certain times and rejecting them at others. Mild coercion and strong encouragement may be necessary in such cases, as well as careful administration of drugs.

Definition and Background of Outpatient Commitment

Many supporters of outpatient commitment believe that the problems of most revolving-door patients would be substantially solved if reasonable constraints were placed on identified noncompliers. Thus, the basic idea of outpatient commitment is that certain chronically mentally ill persons should no longer be released into the community as totally free agents (often with disastrous results) but should be committed to an agency in the community and made subject to conditions that would ensure their ability to sustain themselves and to remain in the community free of frequent decompensations and rehospitalizations.

Outpatient commitment is the logical successor to two earlier trends in mental health law. The first is the procedure of conditional release—an unstructured process in which judges, guided either by ambiguous statutes or acting on their own ill-defined discretion, established certain conditions for the release of patients from mental hospitals. Conditional release has long been a technique for exercising control over discharged criminal offenders who were hospitalized rather than imprisoned because they had been acquitted of criminal charges by reason of insanity. Discharge from a maximum-security mental hospital is typically conditioned on assurances that the released patient will accept medications after discharge (Chan, 1982). Many judges are reluctant, however, to impose such conditions on civil patients. But more and more judges now recognize that certain civil patients require such constraints if they are to be maintained successfully in the community.

Another trend has been the development of the doctrine of the least restrictive or least intrusive alternative, which requires that efficacious care, treatment, and control of the mentally ill be administered in a manner that is least restrictive of their interests in physical freedom and autonomous decision making (Miller and Fiddleman, 1984). There are many state statutes now requiring that, when decisions are to be made that affect the so-called liberty interests of the mentally ill—such as whether to hospitalize, to medicate, or to transfer from one ward to another—this principle must be applied. Community living tends to be far less restrictive than hospitalization. Many observers regard the conditions that are imposed by outpatient commitment, including requirements to accept medications, as less restrictive than the involuntary hospitalizations faced by noncompliant patients.

The formalization of outpatient commitment statutes has resulted from a recognition that, while the initial objectives of conditional release were sound, its structure and enforcement mechanisms were hopelessly inadequate. New standards and procedures were required.

Standards and Procedures of Outpatient Commitment

Who are the mentally ill for whom outpatient commitment is appropriate, and how do we define them? Not all mentally ill persons require the pressure and controls involved in outpatient commitment. Patients committed to outpatient care and made subject to special constraints should be carefully selected so that the net of control is not cast too widely and indiscriminately.

While outpatient commitment statutes vary considerably, all have certain features in common. The typical outpatient statute is designed to apply to those chronically mentally ill persons who should not remain in the hospital because they are capable of being maintained in the community with the help and supervision of family, friends, or agencies and with the use of appropriate treatment, especially antipsychotic medications. Such persons should have demonstrated by repeated noncompliance that, without constraints or controls, they cannot or will not voluntarily accept treatment, either for lack of insight or for other reasons. The most significant feature of outpatient commitment is that it requires that the patient agree to submit to a treatment program recommended by the judge and the community mental health agency and accepted by the judge. While other forms of treatment are of some importance, it is the obligation of the patient to accept antipsychotic medications that is the most crucial requirement.

Standards for outpatient commitment are usually more inclusive than those required for hospitalization. In many states, involuntary hospitalization requires a showing of the patient's present ongoing dangerousness. This is not so with outpatient commitment, which requires only a showing of a likelihood of future dangerousness resulting from a predicted noncompliance. Tennessee's statute (Tennessee Code, 1984), for example, requires a showing that the patient needs control in order to avoid his or her "predictably and imminently becoming an inpatient." North Carolina's statute refers to potential deterioration resulting from predictable noncompliance that would predictably result in the patient being dangerous. An additional requirement in some statutes is a showing that the patient's current mental condition tends to limit or entirely negate his or her ability to make an informed decision about seeking or complying voluntarily with designated treatment.

Outpatient commitment standards thus deal with situations where the patient is at present nondangerous and competent but is likely to become, in the reasonably near future, both dangerous and incompetent if unmedicated. True, future dangerousness, especially in the long term, is generally difficult to predict (Cocozza and Steadman, 1976). But the problem of prediction is significantly reduced and liberty interests are less arbitrarily invaded in specific cases where the past behavior of the patient has followed a consistent pattern of noncompliance that has invariably resulted in decompensation and subsequent dangerousness. Dangerousness, in these cases, includes dysfunctionality that threatens the physical and emotional well-being of the patient and is not limited just to physical violence (Brooks, 1984).

Similar considerations apply to competence. Patients, when stabilized by the action of antipsychotic medications, may become competent in the sense that they reasonably understand their illness and have insight into the role of drugs in their restoration. But, for persistently noncompliant patients, such competence is short-lived. Thus, too much importance should not be placed on the short-term competence of such patients.

These more inclusive standards for outpatient commitment seem justified by the benefit to the patient of being in the community and free of the restrictions of an institution.

In states without outpatient commitment, the judge normally has only two options: hospitalization or unconditional release. In outpatient commitment states, the judge now has a third option but one that should be exercised only if the mentally ill person is a true revolving-door patient. Moreover, in states with more well-developed statutes, outpatient commitment is not ordered unless the community mental health agency has a treatment program available for the patient, is willing to accept him or her, and the patient is willing to comply with the treatment program. Thus, controls and constraints are imposed only on condition that appropriate services will be made available, and not otherwise. Outpatient commitment would be inappropriate, even hazardous in some cases, if the judge were dissatisfied with the prospective cooperation of the community mental health agency.

The commitment to outpatient treatment is time limited, the usual period being ninety days with permissible extensions. Some outpatients may be able to demonstrate by the nature of their compliance during the first ninety-day period that they no longer need constraints. If so, they should be released from outpatient commitment.

While all candidates for outpatient commitment receive hearings, in some states these procedures are less protective than for hospital commitments. In North Carolina, for example, the patient does not have the right to a state-paid lawyer nor the right to cross-examine the doctor who testifies in his or her case. Both of these are rights traditionally provided at hospitalization hearings. The justification offered by the North Carolina legislature is that such protections are very expensive for the state and withheld here because the restrictions on liberty involved are much less serious. Libertarians are critical of such relaxations of due-process protection.

A significant problem in outpatient commitment is that enforcement of conditions is difficult. Since outpatient commitment patients are by definition noncompliant, techniques must be established to ensure compliance. Concern about successfully managing such noncompliance accounts for much judicial reluctance to take full advantage of outpatient commitment. A judge hates to wake up in the morning and read in the newspaper that a patient he or she released has just killed someone.

Many outpatients become recalcitrant and refuse to report in or take their medications. States respond variously to such challenges. North Carolina's enforcement provisions minimize compulsion. If the outpatient becomes noncompliant, the doctor is required only to make "all reasonable efforts" to solicit compliance. If the patient remains noncompliant, the doctor can ask a sheriff to take the patient into custody and bring him or her to the treatment center for an examination and further persuasion. If the patient still continues to be noncompliant, the doctor can decide either to let him or her alone and later file a petition for hospitalization if the patient engages in dangerous behavior or return the patient to court for a judicial review of the reasons for noncompliance. Choosing to let the patient alone might reflect the doctor's view that nonadherence to medications will not automatically result in a relapse but that closer monitoring might be necessary.

The North Carolina statute does not have stricter enforcement provisions because the legislature believed that noncompliance could normally be overcome by the authority of a court order, by the availability of a sheriff to pick up the patient and bring him or her to the mental health center, and by the attention given to the patient by mental health personnel. Where North Carolina community mental health centers have tried in good faith to make outpatient commitment work, these views have been vindicated, and noncompliance has been overcome (Hiday and Scheid-Cook, 1986). But some centers have not cooperated, and many judges prefer stricter enforcement. In fact, some North Carolina judges prefer not to use outpatient commitment because their statute has no teeth.

Some states do have more rigorous enforcement provisions. A new Kansas statute provides that, if the outpatient refuses to comply with the requirements of the judicial order, the mental health facility that has accepted him or her must immediately report the noncompliance to the court, which may then, within its discretion, issue an ex parte order revoking outpatient treatment and requiring immediate commitment to an inpatient facility. If a request for a hearing is not filed within five days, the order becomes final. If a hearing is held, the issue is whether the patient has complied or not. After the hearing, the court may order hospitalization or continued outpatient treatment with different terms and conditions.

Criticisms of Outpatient Commitment

Libertarian objections to outpatient commitment focus on its expanded control over the lives of the mentally ill in the community, reflecting concern that outpatient commitment will be too broadly applied and many mentally ill persons who don't need such controls will be coerced (Mulvey, Geller, and Roth, 1987).

A recent study by Hiday and Scheid-Cook (1986) of outpatient commitment in North Carolina suggests that this concern is not without merit. In some counties, two-fifths of patients committed to outpatient treatment had not had a prior hospitalization; outpatient commitment thus seemed inappropriate if prior hospitalization, rather than clinical judgment or other data, is regarded as essential evidence of noncompliance. Furthermore, over 50 percent of patients committed had shown no indication of prior dangerousness or refusal of medication.

Such applications of the statute suggest that outpatient commitment can be abused as a new way of controlling the mentally ill. A recently published analysis by Schwartz and Costanzo (1987) argues that outpatient commitment "sanctions rather than curtails the deprivation of individual liberties" (p. 1404). Schwartz and Costanzo further contend that outpatient commitment represents "a return to an era when the perceptions of a disability and the professionally determined need for treatment justified compulsory clinical intervention" (p. 1403). Such abuses are not uncontrollable, however. The education of judges and mental health professionals can help to minimize this serious but possibly short-term problem.

Concern about compulsion seems to focus mainly on enforced medications. The argument is made that hospitalized patients have a right to refuse medications but that committed outpatients do not. Research studies show, however, that the right of hospitalized patients to "refuse" is illusory. Only a very small number of hospitalized patients actually refuse medications, and only a tiny proportion of that small number are permitted to remain unmedicated (Brooks, 1987). If the right of a hospitalized patient to refuse is, in fact, only a paper right, then conditioning outpatient treatment on compelled medications does not really deprive the mentally ill person of a significant protection that he or she would otherwise possess.

But the right to refuse does provide another form of protection in the hospital that is important and might be lost in the community. The legal right to refuse almost surely encourages a more careful and less abusive administration of medications in the hospital, which might not be assured in a community mental health center.

There is a risk that unmonitored administration of medications in community mental health facilities could lead to the types of abuses that have been well documented as occurring in hospitals (Brooks, 1980). Outpatients, then, though denied a right to refuse, should be protected by a statutory right to object and the right to a realistic level of participation in their treatment programs. Such participation should include reviews by outside experts that could lead to a reevaluation of the outpatient's medication programs. Antipsychotic medications should be minimized and outpatient commitment must not be seen as a legal device for compulsorily overmedicating a patient.

Enforcement problems generate practical as well as libertarian concerns. Schwartz and Costanzo (1987), in criticizing enforced treatment, sardonically refer to the "scenario of a disabled person being dragged through the street to his therapy appointment or day program" and conclude that "forcing psychiatric treatment is physically difficult, legally questionable, and publicly unacceptable" (p. 1382).

Such a conclusion seems exaggerated. First, recent decisions of the United States Supreme Court expressing deference to psychiatric decision

126

making make it unlikely that any current outpatient commitment statute would be struck down as unconstitutional (Brooks, 1987). Second, public sentiment, influenced by concern about the dumping of the mentally ill, would almost surely support reasonable programs that would result in fewer decompensations and less dangerousness. On the other hand, forcing treatment is, admittedly, physically difficult. Providers in mental hospitals have no problem because institutions are inherently coercive. But, in contrast, mental health professionals in the community stress voluntarism and are reluctant to impose treatment on their patients. These providers are unaccustomed to working with chronically mentally ill patients, preferring clients for whom noncompliance is not typically a problem. By and large, community mental health staff and leadership have little skill, experience, or even willingness to work with the chronically mentally ill, and they fail to understand the need for pressure, constraints, and outreach.

Hiday and Scheid-Cook (1986) found that, in two selected regions of North Carolina, approximately 12 percent and 14 percent, respectively, of all patients were committed to outpatient treatment, while in two other regions the percentages were only 2 percent and 3 percent. They are convinced that outpatient commitment is less successful where mental health center staff and leadership are less concerned with caring for the chronically mentally ill and not knowledgeable about their needs and about statutory provisions. For example, in some centers when clients do not comply with prescribed treatment or fail to meet appointments, staff members make no effort to help the client, automatically recommending to the court that it terminate the outpatient order, thus ensuring failure.

But enforcement problems have become manageable for cooperative leadership and concerned staff. The study by Hiday and Scheid-Cook suggests that there is a high level of success in compliance and enforcement where community facilities are diligent in trying to make outpatient commitment work.

Another practical problem is that community staffs are fearful of legal liability should they neglect to provide adequate treatment or fail to anticipate their clients' dangerous behaviors that might injure themselves or others. Legislatively enacted immunity provisions may reassure providers that they will not be liable for what happens to patients or others except in cases of egregious negligence.

Does Outpatient Commitment Work?

Outpatient commitment is a new legal approach, still developing and not as yet adequately evaluated. A few early studies have indicated that outpatient commitment has not yet fulfilled its promise. This should surprise no one. Various reasons have been given, such as the failure of community center staffs to implement statutory provisions, the lack of clear-cut monitoring and enforcement provisions, and the failure to select appropriate candidates.

Other studies, however, including one done at Saint Elizabeth Hospital in Washington, have indicated that outpatient commitment has been reasonably successful, although problems in implementation persist (Band and others, 1984). Saint Elizabeth Hospital has had the advantage of being both the outpatient and inpatient facility for its patients. It thus provides unusual continuity, since inpatient staff also function as outpatient staff. The chairman of the Mental Health Commission has said that a particular value of the outpatient commitment is that it keeps the family together. The lawyer who represents patients has favored outpatient commitment because it encourages patients to acknowledge their mental problems while recognizing that they can be treated in the community. His only criticism was that Saint Elizabeth psychiatrists tended to emphasize medications to the exclusion of more comprehensive programs aimed at the total rehabilitation of the patient, an observation that runs counter to libertarian objections that the scope of interventions sanctioned by outpatient commitment is too broad.

Hiday and Scheid-Cook (1986) conclude that outpatient commitment "is working with a group of the chronically mentally ill who otherwise would not accept treatment, would become hospitalized, and consequently would experience a greater deprivation of liberty." They are impressed with the number of committed outpatients who had never before stayed in treatment and who had had histories of dangerous episodes and recurrent rehospitalization, who, under outpatient commitment, have complied with treatment and remained stabilized without dangerous behavior for periods exceeding their six-month follow-up. Hiday and Scheid-Cook hypothesize that a major reason for success or lack of it has been the extent to which courts and mental health centers actively support the objectives of outpatient commitment. Where goals have been implemented with skill and good faith, success has been so apparent that previously resistant mental health centers have been won over. There is a reason to believe that the successful operation of outpatient commitment will generate more funding and support from the state and not be a substitute for services, as some libertarians fear.

References

Band, D., Heine, A., Goldfrank, J., Zanni, G., de Veau, L., Wiant, W., and Peele, R. "Outpatient Commitment: A Thirteen-Year Experience." Paper presented at the fifteenth annual meeting of the American Academy of Psychiatry and the Law, Nassau, Bahamas, 1984.
Brooks, A. D. "The Impact of Law on Psychiatric Hospitalization: Onslaught or Imperative Reform?" In S. Halleck (ed.), *Coping with the Legal Onslaught.*

128

New Directions for Mental Health Services, no. 4. San Francisco: Jossey-Bass, 1979.

Brooks, A. D. "The Constitutional Right to Refuse Antipsychotic Medications." *Bulletin of the American Academy of Psychiatry and the Law*, 1980, *8*, 179-221.

Brooks, A. D. "Defining the Dangerousness of the Mentally Ill: Involuntary Civil Commitment." In M. Craft and A. Craft (eds.), *Mentally Abnormal Offenders*. London: Balliere Tindall, 1984.

Brooks, A. D. "The Right to Refuse Antipsychotic Medications: Law and Policy." *Rutgers Law Review*, 1987, *37* (1), 1-39.

Chan, M. "Outpatient Status: Beyond the Term of Commitment." *Pacific Law Journal*, 1982, *13*, 1189-1205.

Cocozza, J. J., and Steadman, H. J. "The Failure of Psychiatric Predictions of Dangerousness: Clear and Convincing Evidence." *Rutgers Law Review*, 1976, *29*, 1084-1101.

Davis, J. "Antipsychotic Drugs." In H. Kaplan and B. Sadock (eds.), *Comprehensive Textbook of Psychiatry*. Vol. 2. Baltimore, Md.: Williams and Wilkins, 1985.

Durham, M. L., and LaFond, J. "The Empirical Consequences and Policy Implications of Broadening the Statutory Criteria for Civil Commitment." *Yale Law and Policy Review*, 1985, *3*, 395-402.

Geller, J. L. "Rights, Wrongs, and the Dilemna of Coerced Community Treatment." *American Journal of Psychiatry*, 1986, *143*, 259-264.

Hiday, V. A., and Scheid-Cook, T. "The North Carolina Experience in Outpatient Commitment: A Critical Appraisal." Paper presented at the eleventh International Congress on Law and Psychiatry, Montreal, Quebec, Canada, June 1986.

Lamb, H. R. "Deinstitutionalization and the Homeless Mentally Ill." *Hospital and Community Psychiatry*, 1984, *35*, 899-907.

Mechanic, D. "The Challenge of Chronic Mental Illness: A Retrospective and Prospective View." *Hospital and Community Psychiatry*, 1986, *37* (9), 891-896.

Miller, R. D., and Fiddleman, P. B. "Outpatient Commitment: Treatment in the Least Restrictive Environment?" *Hospital and Community Psychiatry*, 1984, *35*, 147-151.

Mulvey, E. P., Geller, J. L., and Roth, L. H. "The Promise and Peril of Involuntary Outpatient Commitment." *American Psychologist*, 1987, *42*, 571-584.

Schwartz, S., and Costanzo, C. "Compelling Treatment in the Community: Distorted Doctrines and Violated Values." *Loyola of Los Angeles Law Review*, 1987, *20*, 1329-1429.

Tennessee Code. Ann. § § 33-6-201, 205 (1984, Suppl. 1986).

Treffert, D. A. "The Obviously Ill Patient in Need of Treatment: A Fourth Standard for Civil Commitment." *Hospital and Community Psychiatry*, 1985, *36*, 259-264.

Alexander D. Brooks is the Justice Joseph Weintraub Professor of Law, Rutgers Law School, Newark, New Jersey, and member of the Institute for Health, Health Care Policy, and Aging Research, Rutgers University.

Index

A

Abramowitz, S., 53, 55
Action for Mental Health, 25-27
Aiken, L. H., 10, 11, 73, 75, 79, 114, 115
Alcohol, Drug Abuse, and Mental Health, block grant, 110
Aldrich, H., 63, 68
Alexander, G. J., 88-89, 90
Allard, M. A., 73, 79
Allen, R. E., 54, 57
Altman, H., 66, 68
American Journal of Psychiatry, 20
American Medical Association (AMA), 24-27
American Psychiatric Association (APA), 24-25, 85, 90, 96; pre-World War II, 15; structure of, in 1945, 19-20
American Psychological Association, 96
Anderson, R., 35, 42
Anthony, W. A., 48, 56
Appel, K. E., 24-25, 31
Archer, R., 53, 57
Ashikaga, T., 12
Atay, J. E., 10, 13, 115
Aviram, U., 100, 103
Axilbund, M. T., 88, 89, 90

B

Bachrach, L., 40, 42, 47, 48-49, 52, 56
Bagarozzi, D. A., 65, 66, 67, 69
Baker, F., 61, 63-64, 65, 66, 68, 69
Balint, M., 35, 42
Ball, F.L.J., 71, 79
Band, D., 127
Bardach, E., 75, 79, 99-101, 103
Barrett, S. A., 36, 39, 45
Bassuk, E., 5, 11, 48, 56, 72, 79
Baumohl, J., 40, 44
Bazzouli, G. J., 9, 11
Bean, J., 72, 80
Beard, J. H., 50, 56

Beiser, M., 47, 50, 56
Bell, W., 88, 91
Benham, L., 44
Bennett, D. H., 5, 13
Bergman, H. C., 63, 69
Bergmann, K., 85, 90
Berzon, P., 65, 68
Blazer, D. G., 43
Blenkner, M., 87, 90
Bleuler, M., 4, 11
Bloom, M., 87, 90
Bootzin, R. R., 110, 116
Boswell, P. C., 38, 45
Bowers, R. V., 19, 31
Bowler, M. K., 98, 103
Boyd, J. L., 52, 56
Bradley, V., 79
Brady, J., 6, 11, 77, 79
Breier, A., 12
Broman, C. L., 38-39, 43
Brooks, A. D., 117, 122, 125-126, 127-128
Brooks, G., 12, 103
Brown, B. M., 94, 103
Brown, G. W., 39, 43, 52, 56
Brown, R. L., 38-39, 43
Brownell, A., 52, 58
Bruce, M. L., 38, 39, 43
Buchanan, J. G., 85, 90
Burke, J. D., 44
Burt, M. R., 108, 110, 115
Byers, E. S., 55, 56

C

Calhoun, L., 53, 56
Caragonne, P., 65, 66, 68
Carling, P. J., 76-77, 79
Carstairs, G. M., 52, 56
Case management: case managers and programs in, 65-68; and client advocacy, 64; and confidentiality, 64; and financing care, 114; as formal organization, 61-68; and mental health service systems, 66-68; as primary group, 61-68; role conflict

129

132

Help-seeking behaviors: and age,
39–40; and gender, 38–39; predispos-
ing factors in, 36–41; prevalence of,
34–36; and social class, 37–38; and
social relationships, 40–41; and
substance abusers, 34; variety of,
33–34
Helzer, J. E., 44
Henisz, J. E., 38, 45
Herker, D., 63, 68
Herman, G. H., 99, 104
Hiday, V. A., 124, 126, 127, 128
Hispanics: and help-seeking behav-
ior, 37; and utilization of mental
health services, 41
Hoadley, J. F., 98, 103
Hogan, R., 78, 79, 100, 104
Hogarty, G. E., 55, 57
Hollingshead, A. B., 37, 43
Holzer, C. E., 43
Homelessness, and mental illness, 4–5
Hopper, K., 73, 79
Hopp, M., 64, 70
Horwitz, A. V., 35, 38–39, 39, 41, 43
House Interstate and Foreign Com-
merce Committee, 96
House and Senate Appropriations
Committees, 96
House, J., 52, 57
Housing Act of 1949, 74
Huffine, C. L., 4, 12, 39, 42
Hughes, M., 36, 43
Huxley, P., 35, 37, 40, 41, 43

I

Intagliata, J., 61, 62, 63–64, 66, 69
Integrated Mental Health, Inc., 102
Isaak, A., 94, 104

J

Jackson, B. A., 90
Jaffee, M. W., 90
JCMIH. See Joint Commission on
Mental Illness and Health
Jews, and help-seeking behavior, 37
Johnson, E., 40, 44
Johnson, P. J., 66, 69
Joint Commission on the Accredita-
tion of Hospitals, 62, 69

Joint Commission on Mental Illness
and Health (JCMIH), 31; analyses
and recommendations of, 25–27;
and federal policy, 27–30; work of,
24–27

K

Kadushin, C., 33, 37, 41, 43
Kane, R. A., 86, 90
Kane, R. L., 86, 90
Kanter, J. S., 63, 64–65, 69
Kaplan, H. B., 54, 57
Katz, S., 86, 90
Kay, D.W.K., 85, 90
Keating, D., 73, 77, 79
Keeler, E. B., 9, 12
Keet, M., 41, 43
Keith, S. J., 51, 53, 57
Kemp, B. J., 63–64, 69
Kennedy, J. F., 27–28, 29, 31
Kessler, L. G., 44
Kessler, R. C., 38–39, 43, 52, 54, 57
Kiesler, C. A., 4, 12
Killian, L. M., 36, 45
Kleiner, R. J., 51, 53, 59
Kohn, M., 53, 57
Koyanagi, C., 112–113, 116
Kramer, M., 35, 43
Krieger, M., 42, 44
Kulka, R. A., 36, 37, 38, 39, 45
Kurtz, L. F., 65, 66, 67, 69

L

LaFond, J., 118, 128
Lam, J., 77, 80
Lamb, H. R., 47, 48, 54, 57, 66, 68,
69, 72, 79, 80, 118, 128
Langer, E., 54, 58
Langner, T. S., 44
Lanterman-Petris-Short Act, 100
Lasswell, H. D., 94, 104
Law enforcement, and help-seeking
behaviors, 34, 37, 40
Lazarus, R. S., 54, 56
Leaf, P. J., 35, 38, 39, 40, 43, 44
Leff, J. P., 52, 59
LeGates, R., 73, 77, 79
Leggett, J., 53, 57
Lehman, A., 47, 52, 57, 113, 116
Lerman, P., 36, 43, 101–102, 104

1. TITLE OF PUBLICATION	A. PUBLICATION NO.	2. DATE OF FILING
New Directions for Mental Health Services	4 9 3 - 9 1 0	10/7/87

3. FREQUENCY OF ISSUE	3A. NO. OF ISSUES PUBLISHED ANNUALLY	3B. ANNUAL SUBSCRIPTION PRICE
quarterly	4	$39 indiv/$52 inst

4. COMPLETE MAILING ADDRESS OF KNOWN OFFICE OF PUBLICATION (Street, City, County, State and ZIP Code) (Not printers)

433 California St., San Francisco, San Francisco County, CA 94104

5. COMPLETE MAILING ADDRESS OF THE HEADQUARTERS OR GENERAL BUSINESS OFFICES OF THE PUBLISHERS (Not printers)

433 California St., San Francisco, San Francisco County, CA 94104

6. FULL NAMES AND COMPLETE MAILING ADDRESS OF PUBLISHER, EDITOR, AND MANAGING EDITOR (This item MUST not be blank)

PUBLISHER (Name and Complete Mailing Address)

Jossey-Bass Inc., Publishers, 433 California St., San Francisco CA 94104

EDITOR (Name and Complete Mailing Address)

H. Richard Lamb,1861 Lombardy Rd., San Marino CA 91108

MANAGING EDITOR (Name and Complete Mailing Address)

Allen Jossey-Bass, Jossey-Bass Publishers, 433 California St., SF CA 94104

7. OWNER (If owned by a corporation, its name and address must be stated and also immediately thereunder the names and addresses of stockholders owning or holding 1 percent or more of total amount of stock. If not owned by a corporation, the names and addresses of the individual owners must be given. If owned by a partnership or other unincorporated firm, its name and address, as well as that of each individual must be given. If the publication is published by a nonprofit organization, its name and address must be stated.) (Item must be completed)

FULL NAME	COMPLETE MAILING ADDRESS
Jossey-Bass Inc., Publishers	433 California St., San Francisco CA 94104
for names and addresses of stockholders, see attached list	

8. KNOWN BONDHOLDERS, MORTGAGEES, AND OTHER SECURITY HOLDERS OWNING OR HOLDING 1 PERCENT OR MORE OF TOTAL AMOUNT OF BONDS, MORTGAGES OR OTHER SECURITIES (If there are none, so state)

FULL NAME	COMPLETE MAILING ADDRESS
same as #7	

9. FOR COMPLETION BY NONPROFIT ORGANIZATIONS AUTHORIZED TO MAIL AT SPECIAL RATES (Section 411.3, DMM only)
The purpose, function, and nonprofit status of this organization and the exempt status for Federal income tax purposes (Check one)

☐ (1) HAS NOT CHANGED DURING PRECEDING 12 MONTHS ☐ (2) HAS CHANGED DURING PRECEDING 12 MONTHS (If changed, publisher must submit explanation of change with this statement.)

10. EXTENT AND NATURE OF CIRCULATION	AVERAGE NO. COPIES EACH ISSUE DURING PRECEDING 12 MONTHS	ACTUAL NO. COPIES OF SINGLE ISSUE PUBLISHED NEAREST TO FILING DATE
A. TOTAL NO. COPIES (Net Press Run)	2000	2142
B. PAID CIRCULATION 1. SALES THROUGH DEALERS AND CARRIERS, STREET VENDORS AND COUNTER SALES	271	20
2. MAIL SUBSCRIPTION	1254	1263
C. TOTAL PAID CIRCULATION (Sum of 10B1 and 10B2)	1525	1283
D. FREE DISTRIBUTION BY MAIL, CARRIER OR OTHER MEANS SAMPLES, COMPLIMENTARY AND OTHER FREE COPIES	106	162
E. TOTAL DISTRIBUTION (Sum of C and D)	1631	~1445
F. COPIES NOT DISTRIBUTED 1. OFFICE USE, LEFT OVER, UNACCOUNTED, SPOILED AFTER PRINTING	369	697
2. RETURN FROM NEWS AGENTS		
G. TOTAL (Sum of E, F1 and 2 - should equal net press run shown in A)	2000	2142

11. I certify that the statements made by me above are correct and complete

SIGNATURE AND TITLE OF EDITOR, PUBLISHER, BUSINESS MANAGER OR OWNER

Vice-President

PS Form 3526, July 1981

(See instruction on reverse)

(Page 1)